AACN

American Association of Critical-Care Nurses

Standards for Nursing Care of the Critically Ill

second edition

■   ■   ■   ■   ■   ■   ■   ■   ■

Sarah J. Sanford, R.N., M.A., C.N.A.A.
Senior Vice President
Patient Care Services
Overlake Hospital Medical Center
Bellevue, Washington
Assistant Clinical Professor
School of Nursing
University of Washington
Seattle, Washington

Joanne M. Disch, R.N., Ph.D.
Clinical Director
Department of Medical Nursing, Emergency Services
  and Dialysis
Hospital of the University of Pennsylvania
Associate Professor of Medical Nursing
University of Pennsylvania School of Nursing
Philadelphia, Pennsylvania

APPLETON & LANGE
Norwalk, Connecticut/San Mateo, California

0-8385-0052-8

89 90 91 92 93 / 10 9 8 7 6 5 4 3 2 1

Prentice Hall International (UK) Limited, *London*
Prentice Hall of Australia Pty. Limited, *Sydney*
Prentice Hall Canada, Inc., *Toronto*
Prentice Hall Hispanoamericana, S.A., *Mexico*
Prentice Hall of India Private Limited, *New Delhi*
Prentice Hall of Japan, Inc., *Tokyo*
Simon & Schuster Asia Pte. Ltd., *Singapore*
Editora Prentice Hall do Brasil Ltda., *Rio de Janeiro*
Prentice Hall, *Englewood Cliffs, New Jersey*

Library of Congress Cataloging-in-Publication Data

Sanford, Sarah J.
Standards for nursing care of the critically ill.—2nd ed.
Sarah J. Sanford, Joanne M. Disch.
       p.   cm.
    Rev. ed. of: Standards for nursing care of the critically ill
[developed by the American Association of Critical-Care Nurses].
© 1981.
    "Sponsored by the American Association of Critical–Care Nurses."
    ISBN 0-8385-0052-8
    1. Intensive care nursing—Standards.   2. Intensive care units—
Standards.   I. Disch, Joanne Marilyn.   II. American Association of
Critical–Care Nurses.   III. American Association of Critical-Care
Nurses. Standards for nursing care of the critically ill.
IV. Title.
    [DNLM: 1. Critical Care—standards—nurses' instruction.   WY 154 S217s]
RT 120.I5S26   1989
610.73`61—dc20
DNLM/DLC   89-6558
for Library of Congress   CIP

Production and Design: Chernow Editorial Services, Inc.
Acquisitions Editor: Janet Foltin

Contents

■ ■ ■ ■ ■ ■ ■ ■

List of Tables

■ ■ ■ ■ ■ ■ ■ ■ ■

Preface
■ ■ ■ ■ ■ ■ ■ ■ ■

In 1969, the American Association of Critical-Care Nurses (AACN) was established to improve nursing care to the critically ill by education of critical care nurses. Through the presentation of educational programs, the publication of the *Core Curriculum for Critical Care Nursing* and numerous other books and articles, and the establishment of the certification examination, AACN positively affected the care of critically ill patients and their families.

In 1981, AACN published the first edition of the *Standards for Nursing Care of the Critically Ill*, thus making explicit a set of expectations related to the process by which critical care nurses provided care and controlled the critical care environment. This document was based on Lang's quality assurance model[1] which included the following steps: identify values; identify structure, process, and outcome standards and criteria; secure measurements needed to determine degree of attainment of standards and criteria; make interpretations about strengths and weaknesses based on measurements; identify possible courses of action; choose a course of action and take it. Just as the model was open and circular to indicate its dynamic nature, so too were the standards viewed as dynamic and interactive with the nurses implementing them.

Since that time, the Association and critical care nurses throughout the world have worked to implement the Standards. Incorporating the Standards in daily practice, using them as a framework for educational programming, integrating them into management tools for the evaluation of critical care nursing practice and the critical care environment—these and other uses reflect the ways in which the Standards have influenced the care of the critically ill.

With this second edition, we have retained many of the original statements of standards: generic elements of critical care nursing practice, based on the nursing process, remain largely the same. What has been greatly expanded, however, are the sections targeted toward helping critical care nurses implement the Standards. It has become readily apparent that publication of a document such as the Standards is not enough; implementation of the standards into daily practice is also necessary if the Standards are to have the desired effect on patient care.

Over the years, we have interacted with thousands of critical care nurses committed to providing optimal care to their patients and families—and we

---

[1]Model for Quality Assurance: Implementation of Standards. (Copyright 1975 by the American Nurses Association).

have been tremendously impressed with their commitment and enthusiasm. Moreover, we have come away from the interactions renewed and challenged. It is to these professionals and colleagues that we dedicate this edition.

Sarah J. Sanford
Joanne M. Disch

Acknowledgments

■　　■　　■　　■　　■　　■　　■　　■　　■

By definition, second editions of published works build upon the foundation of the original document. In preparing the second edition of *AACN's Standards for Nursing Care of the Critically Ill*, we were repeatedly aware that the foundation provided by AACN's first standards document remains both comprehensive and relevant. Our most sincere appreciation, therefore, goes to the editors, contributors, and reviewers of the original AACN standards document for providing us such a quality product with which to work.

We are also indebted to the members of the nursing staff of the critical care units at the Hospital of the University of Pennsylvania in Philadelphia and at Overlake Hospital Medical Center in Bellevue, Washington. They willingly shared their experiences, time, and expertise throughout the manuscript development process.

Sarah J. Sanford
Joanne M. Disch

AACN's Definition of Critical Care Nursing

■   ■   ■   ■   ■   ■   ■   ■   ■

In *Nursing, A Social Policy Statement*, the American Nurses' Association defines nursing as "the diagnosis and treatment of human responses to actual or potential health problems." Critical care nursing is that specialty within nursing which deals specifically with human responses to life-threatening problems.

Adopted by AACN Board of Directors,
February 1984

Scope of Critical Care Nursing Practice

■   ■   ■   ■   ■   ■   ■   ■   ■

INTRODUCTION

AACN builds on the ANA definition of nursing[2] and defines critical care nursing as that specialty within nursing which deals with human responses to life threatening problems.[1] The scope of critical care nursing is defined by the dynamic interaction of the critically ill patient, the critical care nurse, and the critical care environment.

The goal of critical care nursing is to ensure effective interaction of these three requisite elements to effect competent nursing practice and optimal patient outcomes within an environment supportive of both. The framework within which critical care nursing is practiced is based on a scientific body of knowledge, the nursing process, and multidisciplinary collaboration in the care of patients.

Although a distinct specialty, critical care nursing is inseparable from the profession of nursing as a whole. As members of the profession, critical care nurses hold the same commitment to protect, maintain, and restore health as well as to embrace the *Code for Nurses*.[3]

THE CRITICALLY ILL PATIENT

Central to the scope of critical care nursing is the critically ill patient who is characterized by the presence of, or being at high risk for developing, life threatening problems. The critically ill patient requires constant intensive, multidisciplinary assessment and intervention in order to restore stability, prevent complications, and achieve and maintain optimal responses.

In recognition of the critically ill patients' primary need for restoration of physiologic stability, the critical care nurse coordinates interventions directed at resolving life-threatening problems. Nursing activities also focus on support of patient adaptation, restoration of health, and preservation of patient rights, including the right to refuse treatment or to die. Inherent in the patients' response to critical illness is the need to maintain psychological, emotional, and social integrity. The familiarity, comfort, and support provided by social relationships can enhance effective coping. Therefore, the concept of the critically ill patient includes the interaction and impact of the patients' family and/ or significant other(s).

THE CRITICAL CARE NURSE

The critical care nurse is a licensed professional who is responsible for ensuring that all critically ill patients receive optimal care. Basic to accomplishment of this goal is individual professional accountability through adherence to standards of nursing care of the critically ill and through a commitment to act in accordance with ethical principles.

Critical care nursing practice encompasses the diagnosis and treatment of patient responses to life threatening health problems. The critical care nurse is the one constant in the critical care environment. As such, coordination of the care delivered by various health care providers is an intrinsic responsibility of the critical care nurse. With the nursing process as a framework, the critical care nurse uses independent, dependent, and interdependent interventions to restore stability, prevent complications, and achieve and maintain optimal patient responses. Independent nursing interventions are those actions which are in the unique realm of nursing and include manipulation of the environment, teaching, counseling, and initiating referrals. Dependent nursing interventions are those actions prescribed by medicine. Interdependent nursing interventions are actions determined through multidisciplinary collaboration. Underlying the application of these interventions is a holistic approach that expresses human warmth and caring. This art, in conjunction with the science of critical care nursing, is essential to the interaction between the critical care nurse and critically ill patient in attaining optimal outcomes.

The critical care environment is constantly changing. The critical care nurse must respond effectively to the demands created by this environment for the broad application of knowledge. Realization of this goal is accomplished through entry preparation into professional nursing practice at a baccalaureate level and a commitment to maintaining competency in critical care nursing through ongoing education concurrent with an expanding base of experience.

THE CRITICAL CARE ENVIRONMENT

The critical care environment can be viewed from three perspectives. On one level the critical care environment is defined by those conditions and circumstances surrounding the direct interaction between the critical care nurse and the critically ill patient. The immediate environment must constantly support this interaction in order to effect desired patient outcomes. Adequate resources, in the form of readily available emergency equipment, needed supplies, effective support systems for managing emergent patient situations, and measures for ensuring patient safety are requisites. The framework for nursing practice in this setting is provided by standards of nursing care of the critically ill.

The institution or setting within which critically ill patients receive care represents another perspective of the critical care environment. At this level, the critical care management and administrative structure ensures effective care delivery systems for various populations of critically ill patients through provision of adequate human, material, and financial resources, through required quality systems, and through maintenance of standards of nursing care of the critically ill.

Additional elements contributing to effective care delivery include:

- Participatory decision-making which ensures that the critical care nurse provides input into decisions affecting the nurse-patient interaction.

- A collaborative practice model that facilitates multidisciplinary problem-solving and ethical decision-making.

- Education of critical care nurses consistent with standards for critical care nursing education and practice.

The broadest perspective of the environment encompasses a global view of those factors that impact the provision of care to the critically ill patient. Monitoring of legal, regulatory, social, economic, and political trends is necessary to promote early recognition of the potential implications for critical care nursing and to provide a basis for a timely response.

REFERENCES:

[1]AACN, "Definition of Critical Care Nursing" AACN Position Statement, February, 1984.
[2]ANA, *Nursing: A Social Policy Statement*, ANA, Kansas City, Missouri, 1980.
[3]ANA, *Code for Nurses, ANA, Kansas City, Missouri, 1985.*
(Adopted by AACN Board of Directors, November 1986)

P·A·R·T I

Introduction

■   ■   ■   ■   ■   ■   ■   ■

▪
context
▪

Quality of care is a multidimensional, yet elusive, concept that reflects a judgment about the level of care rendered to a patient. One way to quantify a particular level of care and, thus, provide a mechanism for measuring its attainment is to establish standards. Standards are statements of quality which serve as a model to facilitate and evaluate the delivery of care. Historically, society has delegated the establishment of standards regarding professional practice to the professions. Indeed, one of the elements defining a profession is that it establishes and enforces its own standards.

The delivery of quality care to the critically ill has been a primary goal of the American Association of Critical-Care Nurses (AACN) since its inception in 1969. To that end, the first edition of the *Standards for Nursing Care of the Critically Ill* was published in 1980, affording a framework for both practice and evaluation of care provided to critically ill individuals and their families.

Since that time, the health care environment within which critical care nursing is practiced has radically changed. High costs, limited resources, and increasing demand have combined to increase emphasis on the efficiency and cost-effectiveness of all areas of health care service delivery. While quality is still a primary concern, the role that consumer groups, regulatory agencies, and public and private institutions play in monitoring the process of care delivery and the outcomes of care has increased. Consequently, the province of quality assessment and assurance has extended beyond professional self-regulation into other areas. Nonetheless, accountability for defining standards of practice remains with the profession.

Critical care nursing is the diagnosis and treatment of human responses to actual or potential life-threatening illness. From this definition, the scope of practice of critical care nursing is derived. This scope reflects a triad, incorporating the concepts of the critically ill patient, the critical care nurse, and an environment supportive of the care of the critically ill (see American Association of Critical-Care Nurses Scope of Critical Care Nursing Practice, p. xv). For there to be optimal outcomes, all three factors must be addressed. Because the scope refers to the patient, nurse, and environment, the method for quality assurance espoused by Donabedian (1968) provides direction for the development of standards for the care of the critically ill.

▪
conceptual
framework
▪

Developed in the 1960s, this model posits that a comprehensive evaluation of care encompasses consideration of three factors. First, the process of care delivery must be examined, i.e., elements of professional practice, such as assessment, diagnosis, planning, implementation, and evaluation. Standards by which the process of care is appraised are developed by leaders within the profession and reflect appropriate care delivery for specific patient situations. Thus, the focus for evaluation here is the practitioner and the appropriateness, competence, and technical correctness of interventions provided.

The second factor to be considered is the outcome or end result of the process. In some situations, the purpose for evaluation is not to determine whether the process was sufficient or appropriate, but whether it was effective or resulted in the desired impact or outcome. While outcomes of health care are difficult to define and measure, the use of this patient-centered criterion has captured a great deal of attention over the past few years.

A third factor which provides indirect information for evaluation of the quality of patient care can be obtained through consideration of the degree to which the environment supports or facilitates therapeutic interventions (structures and settings which support and surround the process of care). In this context, structure includes the physical aspects of facilities and equipment as well as the characteristics of the resources used to provide care and the manner in which they are organized. It must be pointed out, however, that characteristics such as practitioner qualifications and organizational structure are not necessarily themselves equated with a quality outcome, nor do they guarantee quality. Rather, Donabedian suggests that a relationship exists between their existence and quality outcomes.

Use of a framework composed of several dimensions for the evaluation of quality is essential for a concept characterized earlier as multidimensional and elusive. The composite assessment obtained when all three factors are considered simultaneously is greater than the sum of the parts since interrelationships certainly exist among them. Moreover, this framework is particularly applicable to the care of the critically ill. The scope of critical care nursing practice is a function of a knowledgeable and competent professional, prepared within the specialty of critical care nursing practice; a critically ill patient and family; and an environment which is suitably equipped with the necessary resources. This latter component allows for the care of critically ill patients by appropriately prepared individuals in other than geographically delineated intensive care units. In other words, both the scope of practice as defined by AACN and Donabedian's framework acknowledge that critical care nursing need not be limited to specific units but occurs when the requisite elements are present (i.e., a critically ill patient can attain quality outcomes when cared for on a general care unit with sufficient supportive resources, among them a competent critical care nurse).

The second edition of the *Standards for Nursing Care of the Critically Ill* presents process and structure standards (Parts II and III) related to the care of the critically ill. Recently, AACN has embarked upon an ambitious project to identify patient-centered outcome standards relevant to this same population. Upon their completion, the three components of Donabedian's model for quality assurance—structure, process, and outcome standards—will be integrated and available for application to the care of critically ill individuals.

   In the meantime, this book includes content designed to assist critical care nurses in using the process standards to develop specific outcome standard statements. Part IV describes the implementation of the standards and will aid clinicians, educators, and managers in concretely using the standards. Additionally, this edition of the *Standards* presents examples of compliance with individual process standards. To be emphasized throughout is the dynamic nature of the processes of developing standards for and evaluating the care of the critically ill.

REFERENCES

AACN. (1986). *Scope of Critical Care Nursing Practice*. Newport Beach, CA: AACN.
Donabedian, A. (1968). *Bull. N.Y. Acad. Med.*, *44*(2), Feb 1968, 117–124.

P·A·R·T II

Process Standards

■ ■ ■ ■ ■ ■ ■ ■

■ ——————— **VALUE STATEMENT** ——————— ■

The critical care nurse shall utilize the nursing process in the delivery of patient care.

■ ————————————————————————————— ■

I. Comprehensive Standard: Data shall be collected continuously on all critically ill patients wherever they may be located.

I.a. *Supporting Standard*: The critical care nurse shall collect subjective and objective data to determine the gravity of the patient's problems/needs.

I.b. *Supporting Standard*: The critical care nurse shall collect subjective and objective data within a time period which reflects the gravity of the patient's problems/needs.

I.c. *Supporting Standard*: The critical care nurse shall collect data in an organized, systematic fashion to ensure completeness of assessment.

I.d. *Supporting Standard*: The critical care nurse shall utilize appropriate physical examination techniques.

I.e. *Supporting Standard*: The critical care nurse shall demonstrate technical competency in gathering objective data.

I.f. *Supporting Standard*: The critical care nurse shall demonstrate competency in communication skills.

I.g. *Supporting Standard*: The critical care nurse shall gather pertinent social and psychological data from the patient, significant others, and other health team members.

I.h. *Supporting Standard*: The critical care nurse shall collect pertinent data from previous patient records.

I.i. *Supporting Standard*: The critical care nurse shall collaborate with other health team members to collect data.

I.j. *Supporting Standard*: The critical care nurse shall facilitate the availability of pertinent data to all health team members.

I.k. *Supporting Standard*: The critical care nurse shall revise the data base as new information is available.

I.l. *Supporting Standard*: The critical care nurse shall document all pertinent data in the patient's record.

II. Comprehensive Standard: The identification of patient problems/needs and their priority shall be based upon collected data.

II.a. *Supporting Standard*: The critical care nurse shall utilize collected data to establish a list of actual and potential patient problems/needs.

II.b. *Supporting Standard*: The critical care nurse shall collaborate with the patient, significant others, and other health team members in identification of problems/needs.

II.c. *Supporting Standard*: The critical care nurse shall utilize collected data to formulate hypotheses as to the etiologic bases for each identified actual or potential problem/need.

II.d. *Supporting Standard*: The critical care nurse shall utilize nursing diagnoses for the actual or potential problems/needs which nurses, by virtue of education and experience, are able, responsible, and accountable to treat.

II.e. *Supporting Standard*: The critical care nurse shall establish the priority of problems/needs according to the actual/potential threat to the patient.

II.f. *Supporting Standard*: The critical care nurse shall reassess the list of actual or potential problems/needs and their priority as the data base changes.

II.g. *Supporting Standard*: The critical care nurse shall record identified actual or potential problems/needs, indicating priority, in the patient's record.

III. Comprehensive Standard: An appropriate plan of nursing care shall be formulated.

   III.a. *Supporting Standard*: The critical care nurse shall develop the plan of care in collaboration with the patient, significant others, and other health team members.

   III.b. *Supporting Standard*: The critical care nurse shall determine nursing interventions for each problem/need.

   III.c. *Supporting Standard*: The critical care nurse shall incorporate interventions that communicate acceptance of the patient's beliefs, culture, religion, and socioeconomic background.

   III.d. *Supporting Standard*: The critical care nurse shall identify areas for education of the patient and significant others.

   III.e. *Supporting Standard*: The critical care nurse shall develop appropriate goals for each problem/need in collaboration with the patient, significant others, and other health team members.

   III.f. *Supporting Standard*: The critical care nurse shall organize the plan to reflect the priority of identified problems/needs.

   III.g. *Supporting Standard*: The critical care nurse shall revise the plan of care to reflect the patient's current status.

   III.h. *Supporting Standard*: The critical care nurse shall identify activities through which care will be evaluated.

   III.i. *Supporting Standard*: The critical care nurse shall communicate the plan to those involved in the patient's care.

   III.j. *Supporting Standard*: The critical care nurse shall record the plan of nursing care in the patient record.

IV. Comprehensive Standard: The plan of nursing care shall be implemented according to the priority of identified problems/needs.

IV.a. *Supporting Standard*: The critical care nurse shall implement the plan of nursing care in collaboration with the patient, significant others, and other health team members.

IV.b. *Supporting Standard*: The critical care nurse shall support and promote patient participation in care.

IV.c. *Supporting Standard*: The critical care nurse shall deliver care in an organized, humanistic manner.

IV.d. *Supporting Standard*: The critical care nurse shall integrate current scientific knowledge with technical and psychomotor competency.

IV.e. *Supporting Standard*: The critical care nurse shall provide care in such a way as to prevent complications and life-threatening situations.

IV.f. *Supporting Standard*: The critical care nurse shall coordinate care delivered by other health team members.

IV.g. *Supporting Standard*: The critical care nurse shall document interventions in the record.

V. Comprehensive Standard: The results of nursing care shall be continuously evaluated.

> **V.a.** *Supporting Standard*: The critical care nurse shall assure the relevance of nursing interventions to identified patient problems/needs.
>
> **V.b.** *Supporting Standard*: The critical care nurse shall collect data for evaluation within an appropriate time interval after intervention.
>
> **V.c.** *Supporting Standard*: The critical care nurse shall compare the patient's response with expected results.
>
> **V.d.** *Supporting Standard*: The critical care nurse shall base the evaluation on data from pertinent sources.
>
> **V.e.** *Supporting Standard*: The critical care nurse shall collaborate with the patient, significant others, and other health team members in the evaluation process.
>
> **V.f.** *Supporting Standard*: The critical care nurse shall attempt to determine the cause of any significant differences between the patient's response and the expected response.
>
> **V.g.** *Supporting Standard*: The critical care nurse shall review the plan of care and revise it based on the evaluation results.
>
> **V.h.** *Supporting Standard*: The critical care nurse shall document evaluation findings in the patient record.

BIBLIOGRAPHY

AACN. (1981). *Standards for Nursing Care of the Critically Ill.* Thierer, J., et al. (eds.). Reston, VA: Reston Publishing Company.

Alspach, J., et al. (eds.). (1985). *AACN's Core Curriculum for Critical Care Nursing* (3rd ed.). St. Louis: C. V. Mosby.

Carpenito, L. J. (1987). *Nursing Diagnosis Application to Clinical Practice* (2nd ed.). Philadelphia: J. B. Lippincott.

Hazinski, M. F. (1984). *Nursing Care of the Critically Ill Child.* St. Louis: C. V. Mosby.

Joint Commission on Accreditation of Healthcare Organizations. (1987). *Accreditation Manual for Hospitals/88.* Chicago: Joint Commission.

Kinney, M., et al. (eds.). (1988). *AACN's Clinical Reference for Critical Care Nursing* (2nd ed.). New York: McGraw Hill.

Millar, S., et al. (eds.). (1985). *AACN Procedure Manual for Critical Care* (2nd ed.). Philadelphia: W. B. Saunders.

P•A•R•T III

Structure Standards

■　■　■　■　■　■　■　■

■ ———————————— **VALUE STATEMENT** ———————————— ■

The critical care nurse shall be cognizant of and have concern for those factors which ensure a safe and effective environment in which care to the critically ill is delivered.

■ ——— ■

I. **Comprehensive Standard:** The critical care unit shall be designed to ensure a safe and supportive environment for critically ill patients and for the personnel who care for them.

I.a. *Supporting Standard*: The critical care nurse shall participate in the development of the philosophy of use, and in the designing and planning of new or renovated critical care units.

I.b. *Supporting Standard*: The critical care nurse shall be cognizant of various rules and/or regulations governing physical facilities for care of critically ill patients, such as those established by the:

- city

- state

- Department of Health and Human Services

- Joint Commission on Accreditation of Healthcare Organizations

I.c. *Supporting Standard*: The critical care nurse shall ensure that the patient's privacy is protected without losing constant surveillance capability through the planning and design of the unit:

- adequate space per patient bed, with consideration of potential equipment needs

- adequate electrical outlets

- adequate illumination

- windows, clocks, calendars

- plumbing/sewage and sinks

- use of proper colors for walls, ceilings, and furnishings

- use of acoustic materials to minimize noise

- life-support systems, including medical gases, suction outlets, and emergency power availability

- adequate space for support areas, including but not limited to:

  - nursing station

  - office space

  - clean and soiled utility areas

  - linen storage

  - equipment storage

  - medication room

  - janitor's closet

  - visitors' waiting area

  - conference room

  - staff lounge area

  - nourishment station

  - emergency equipment storage

  - adequate ventilation and humidity/temperature control individualized for each patient room

I.d. *Supporting Standard*: The critical care nurse shall ensure that a communication system within the unit provides for:

- routine patient care

- notification of appropriate personnel in emergencies

I.e. *Supporting Standard*: The critical care nurse shall ensure that the monitoring systems are appropriate such that patient condition and needs for monitoring and privacy are considered.

I.f. *Supporting Standard*: The critical care nurse shall be cognizant of the radiation hazards present in the critical care environment and shall institute measures to minimize untoward effects on patients, visitors, and personnel. These measures may include:

- development of guidelines for protecting personnel and patients from radiation exposure

- provision of lead shields to be worn by patients and/or personnel during radiologic diagnostic procedures

- periodic examination of the integrity of radiation-related equipment

I.g. *Supporting Standard*: The critical care nurse shall monitor sensory stimuli (e.g., noise, light) and institute measures to facilitate a therapeutic balance.

II. **Comprehensive Standard:** The critical care unit shall be constructed, equipped, and operated in a manner which protects patients, visitors, and personnel from electrical hazards.

II.a. *Supporting Standard*: The critical care unit construction, equipment, and operation shall comply with:

- applicable building codes

- state and/or federal occupational safety and health codes or standards

- current Life Safety Codes of the National Life Protection Association

II.b. *Supporting Standards*: A member of the critical care nursing staff shall participate in the selection of new equipment which will be used in the critical care area.

Instruction by the vendor in the use of new equipment shall be included as part of the purchase agreement. All electrical equipment and/or electronic systems used within critical care shall be inspected for reliable and safe performance. Such inspection shall:

- be performed by a qualified person

- occur prior to initial use, after repair, and thereafter at least semiannually

- be documented

II.c. *Supporting Standard*: Resource persons shall be available to the critical care staff at all times to provide advice and/or service on electrical equipment and electronic systems.

II.d. *Supporting Standard*: Information regarding the use and care of all equipment shall be readily available to the critical care staff.

II.e. *Supporting Standard*: Written policies and procedures regarding electrical safety shall be established. Such policies and procedures shall include, but not be limited to:

- preventive maintenance programs

- general precautions in the care of patients requiring the use of electrically operated devices

- precautions in the care of patients who are particularly prone to electrical hazards, such as those with:

- debilitating conditions

- loss of skin resistance

- indwelling conductive catheters or cardiac leads
- severe electrolyte imbalance
- proper grounding
- restrictions on the use of extension cords and adapters
- inspection and use of patient-owned electrically operated equipment
- prevention of overload to any electrical system
- inspection of electrical equipment and electronic systems
- disposition and servicing of malfunctioning equipment
- regulation and maintenance of appropriate temperature and humidity to prevent electrical hazard.

II.f.   *Supporting Standard*: The critical care nurse shall demonstrate knowledge of and responsibility for implementation of an electrically safe environment and one which is consistent with established policy and procedure.

III. **Comprehensive Standard:** The critical care unit shall be constructed, equipped, and operated in a manner which protects patients, visitors, and personnel from fire hazard.

III.a. *Supporting Standard*: The critical care unit construction, equipment, and operation shall comply with:

- applicable building codes

- fire prevention codes

- state and/or federal occupational safety and health codes or standards

- current Life Safety Codes of the National Fire Protection Association

III.b. *Supporting Standard*: A manually operated fire alarm system shall be available within the critical care unit.

III.c. *Supporting Standard*: Fire extinguishers shall be available within the critical care unit at all times and shall be:

- of the type required for the classes of fire anticipated in the critical care area

- located so as to be readily available when needed

- inspected at least quarterly with the inspection documented

III.d. *Supporting Standard*: A member of the Critical Care Committee shall be a member of the Hospital Safety Committee.

III.e. *Supporting Standard*: The Critical Care Committee shall ensure that policies and procedures which will minimize fire hazards to patients, visitors, and personnel are established and reviewed annually. Such policies and procedures shall include, but not be limited to:

- prevention of fire hazards in the presence of an oxygen-enriched atmosphere

- use, storage, and transportation of gas cylinders

- fire drills

- fire extinguishing system

- evacuation plan

- reporting of fire safety policy violations

- protection of patient records

- orientation and continuing education regarding fire safety practices

III.f.   *Supporting Standard*: Fire drills shall be held at least quarterly for each shift, their occurrence documented and evaluated, and corrective action taken for any deficiency.

III.g.   *Supporting Standard*: The critical care nurse shall demonstrate knowledge of and responsibility for implementation of all aspects of the fire safety program.

IV. **Comprehensive Standard:** The critical care nurse shall have essential equipment, services, and supplies immediately available at all times.

IV.a. *Supporting Standard*: The critical care nurse shall participate in establishing an inventory of necessary equipment and supplies for each unit which will:

- include routine as well as emergency equipment

- reflect the specific needs of the potential patient population

- be reviewed annually

IV.b. *Supporting Standard*: The critical care nurse shall participate in establishing written policies and procedures for ordering, monitoring, and replacing equipment, medication, and supplies needed for each unit.

IV.c. *Supporting Standard*: The critical care nurse shall ensure that equipment, medications, and supplies considered necessary during emergency situations shall:

- be centrally located and readily accessible

- have documented inspection once each shift and after each use by appropriate personnel

IV.d. *Supporting Standard*: The critical care nurse shall be responsible for ensuring the availabilty of necessary supplies and equipment before admission of a new patient.

IV.e. *Supporting Standard*: Provision shall be made for replenishment of needed supplies on a 24-four hour basis.

IV.f. *Supporting Standard*: The critical care nurse shall have knowledge of and access to available clinical and laboratory services that may be necessary during emergency situations.

IV.g. *Supporting Standard*: The critical care nurse shall demonstrate knowledge of and responsibility for obtaining necessary equipment, medications, and supplies.

V. **Comprehensive Standard:** The critical care unit shall have a comprehensive infection control program.

V.a. *Supporting Standard*: Written infection control policies and procedures specific to the unit shall be established and shall comply with any requirements directed by:

- national, state, and local agencies

- Hospital Infection Control Committee

- physical layout of the unit

V.b. *Supporting Standard*: Written infection control policies and procedures shall address the prevention and control of infection among patients, personnel, and visitors. These shall include, but not be limited to:

- patient eligibility for admission, including requirements for equipment and personnel

- methods employed in the prevention of potential nosocomial infections

- storage, handling, and disposal of supplies, waste, and equipment

- control of traffic (hospital personnel and visitors) in the critical care unit and isolation areas

- inspection for outdated sterile items

- environmental disinfection and equipment sterilization

- nursing personnel assignment

- apparel worn by hospital personnel

- specific indications for isolation/precaution requirements in relation to potential or actual diagnosis

- responsibility and authority for initiating and enforcing infection control

- acceptable ventilation patterns, air exchange rates, air temperature, and humidity

V.c. *Supporting Standard*: The Critical Care Committee, in collaboration with the Hospital Infection Control Committee, shall annually review and revise the unit's infection control policies and procedures.

V.d. *Supporting Standard*: The Critical Care Committee and the Hospital Infection Control Committee shall devise an ongoing system for reporting, reviewing, and evaluating infections within the critical care unit.

V.e. *Supporting Standard*: The Critical Care Committee shall monitor all findings from any concurrent and retrospective patient care evaluations that relate to infection control activities within the critical care unit.

V.f. *Supporting Standard*: The quality of patient care shall be maintained regardless of the patient's need for isolation.

V.g. *Supporting Standard*: The Critical Care Committee, in collaboration with the Hospital Infection Control Committee, shall implement a program which will minimize the risk of infection to critical care unit personnel. The components of such a program shall include, but not be limited to:

- the prevention, monitoring, and management of needle stick injuries

- the provision of an immunization program for high-risk health care personnel

- provision of education and material resources needed for the implementation of Universal Precautions

V.h. *Supporting Standard*: The critical care unit orientation shall include:

- introduction to the institution's infection control program

- individual responsibilities for prevention and control of infection

V.i. *Supporting Standard*: Documented inservice education shall be provided at least annually concerning current infection control practices.

V.j. *Supporting Standard*: The critical care nurse shall demonstrate:

- knowledge of the classifications of infectious conditions requiring isolation or precaution

- responsibility for implementation of infection control policies and procedures

V.k. *Supporting Standard*: Infection control resources shall be readily available.

VI. Comprehensive Standard: The critical care unit shall be managed in a manner which ensures the delivery of safe and effective care to the critically ill.

VI.a.   *Supporting Standard*: The critical care unit shall have a written philosophy and objectives which

- reflect the nursing service philosophy and objectives

- guide the nursing activities of the unit

VI.b.   *Supporting Standard*: The operations of the unit shall conform to local, state, and federal laws.

VI.c.   *Supporting Standard*: The critical care nurse shall participate in establishing standards of practice for nursing care.

VI.d.   *Supporting Standard*: The activities of the critical care unit shall be under the direction of a multidisciplinary committee, with appropriate representation from the medical and nursing staffs and other support services directly involved with the critically ill patient.

VI.e.   *Supporting Standard*: The supervision of nursing care in the unit is provided by a registered nurse who has relevant education, training, and experience and who has demonstrated current competence in management.

VI.f.   *Supporting Standard*: A policy and procedures manual shall be developed, annually reviewed, and approved by the Critical Care Committee, subject to approval by the hospital administration. Where appropriate, other nonnursing departments shall participate in the development of these policies and procedures. These shall include, but not be limited to:

- patient admission and discharge criteria

- use of standing orders

- decision-making roles of staff

- evaluation methods to determine the effectiveness of the unit

- ongoing requirements for continuing education of the professional staff

- regulation of visitors

- regulations for traffic control

- safety practices for patients, staff, and visitors

- role of the unit in hospital disaster plans

- procedures for maintenance and repair of equipment

- patient care procedures, including specification of personnel to perform these procedures
- housekeeping procedures
- infection control measures
- list of necessary equipment for the unit
- electrical safety regulations
- fire safety regulations
- medication administration
- patient consultation and referral mechanisms
- discharge planning
- patient and family teaching
- documentation of nursing care given
- maintenance of required records, reports, or statistical information
- scope of activity of volunteers or paid attendants
- initiation of life-sustaining measures
- withholding of resuscitative measures
- termination of life-sustaining measures
- routine inquiry related to tissue and organ donation
- protocols for handling emergency situations

VI.g. *Supporting Standard*: The nursing director of the critical care unit shall work collaboratively with the medical director to assure optimal functioning of the unit.

VI.h. *Supporting Standard*: The critical care unit budget shall be developed and administered by the medical and nursing directors.

VI.i. *Supporting Standard*: The critical care unit shall have a mechanism established for the ongoing monitoring and evaluation of resources used in the provision of care to the critically ill.

VII. Comprehensive Standard: The critical care unit shall have appropriately qualified staff to provide care on a 24-hour basis.

VII.a.   *Supporting Standard*: Members of the professional nursing staff shall possess the following qualifications:

• current registered nurse license

• demonstrated competency in requisite skills

• patient-centered philosophy

• problem-solving ability

• ability to practice within a standards-based format

VII.b.   *Supporting Standard*: Potential staff shall be interviewed and selected by the critical care nurse manager for appropriateness of employment.

VII.c.   *Supporting Standard*: All professional nursing staff shall demonstrate knowledge of and responsibility for the implementation of the unit's policies and procedures.

VII.d.   *Supporting Standard*: There shall be sufficient professional nursing personnel to provide safe, effective patient care. The nurse-patient ratio shall reflect recognition of the patient's acuity and required nursing care. Staffing patterns shall be reviewed regularly by the Critical Care Committee to ensure the delivery of safe care.

VII.e.   *Supporting Standard*: Unit staff shall participate in the development of staffing patterns. These patterns shall provide for:

• the flexibility to give optimum patient care on a 24-hour basis

• utilization of at least a 50% RN staff on each shift

• adequate supervision of other licensed and unlicensed personnel who are delivering direct nursing care

• provisions for unit staff to function intermittently in a support role in other areas, but guaranteeing prompt return to their primary unit when needed

• contingency plans to ensure availability of qualified critical care nursing staff

VII.f.   *Supporting Standard*: Staffing levels will be derived from the utilization of a patient classification system which reflects the full range of nursing functions.

VII.g.   *Supporting Standard*: There shall be ongoing monitoring of productivity levels according to hospital standards.

VIII. Comprehensive Standard: The critical care nurse shall be competent and current in critical care nursing.

VIII.a. *Supporting Standard*: There will be a structured orientation program which will include sufficient didactic and clinical content, as well as the assignment of a clinical preceptor to work closely with the new practitioners in critical care nursing.

VIII.b. *Supporting Standard*: The orientation period will be of a sufficient length to enable beginning practitioners to:

- provide safe, minimal levels of care

- identify human responses commonly encountered in the critically ill

- identify self-limitations and available resources

VIII.c. *Supporting Standard*: Prior to assuming independent responsibility for patient care, the critical care nurse shall demonstrate possession of the knowledge base requisite for the care of the critically ill. This knowledge base shall include that content necessary for:

- collection and processing of data related to the physiological and psychosocial status of the critically ill person

- identification and determination of the priority of the patient's problems/needs

- development of a plan of nursing care

- implementation of the plan of nursing care

- evaluation of care delivered

VIII.d. *Supporting Standard*: Prior to assuming independent responsibility for patient care, the critical care nurse shall demonstrate possession of psychomotor skills common to and requisite for care of the critically ill.

VIII.e. *Supporting Standard*: Prior to assuming independent responsibility for patient care, the critical care nurse shall demonstrate in supervised clinical practice the ability to integrate knowledge and psychomotor skills through applications of the nursing process and subsequent documentation.

VIII.f. *Supporting Standard*: Prior to assuming independent responsibility for patient care, the critical care nurse shall demonstrate possession of sufficient interpersonal skills so as to therapeutically interact with patients and families.

VIII.g. *Supporting Standard*: Critical care nurses shall be responsible for seeking educational resources and creating learning experiences necessary for the achievement and maintenance of currency in their areas of practice. Such experiences may include, but not be limited to:

- independent study

- nursing preceptorship

- inservice classes and grand rounds

- formal orientation

- academic classes

- seminars and symposiums

- rotating assignments under supervision

- affiliation with another institution for a specific learning objective

- tutoring by a nurse consultant

- patient rounds with members of other disciplines

VIII.h. *Supporting Standard*: Additional knowledge and skills shall be required prior to assuming responsibility for the care of patient populations for which the nurse has not been prepared. Characteristics of a patient population to consider when evaluating one's ability to provide care to a new patient population include:

- disease modality

- treatment modality

- age of patient

- acuity

VIII.i. *Supporting Standard*: Responsibility for nursing care is retained by the hospital nursing staff when nursing students and nursing personnel from outside sources provide care in the unit.

VIII.j. *Supporting Standard*: Nursing students will provide care to patients under the guidance and direction of an appropriately prepared nursing staff member or instructor.

VIII.k. *Supporting Standard*: A formal process shall be established for the identification, monitoring, and rehabilitation of the impaired critical care nurse.

VIII.l. *Supporting Standard*: Education/training programs for nursing personnel are ongoing and designed to assist the practitioner in maintaining competency in critical care nursing.

VIII.m. *Supporting Standard*: Critical clinical competencies will be identified, and a mechanism for annual review will be established.

IX. Comprehensive Standard: The critical care nurse's performance appraisal shall be based upon the roles and responsibilities identified in the position description.

IX.a. *Supporting Standard*: Job descriptions shall be criterion-based, written, and readily available for each classification of nursing personnel, and shall include:

- position title

- organizational relationships

- basic functions and responsibilities

- qualifications and special skills needed

- expectations for continuing education

IX.b. *Supporting Standard*: Nursing staff shall be evaluated at the end of the orientation period, at the end of the probationary period, and at least yearly thereafter, or as needed.

IX.c. *Supporting Standard*: The critical care nurse shall actively participate in his/her performance appraisal and in the development of an appropriate plan of action.

IX.d. *Supporting Standard*: A process for peer evaluation shall be established which ensures the provision of constructive feedback.

X. **Comprehensive Standard:** The critical care unit shall have an explicit, systematic, and ongoing program to evaluate care of the critically ill.

X.a. *Supporting Standard*: Criteria for a program for the evaluation of care shall reflect current scientific knowledge, professional values, and relevant regulatory standards.

X.b. *Supporting Standard*: The evaluation program shall include:

- identified standards of care

- ongoing collection of data pertinent to the care of the critically ill

- use of objective, measurable criteria

- regularly scheduled reviews of the data to determine problems

- documented plan of action

- evaluation of the effectiveness of the plan of action

XI. **Comprehensive Standard:** Critical care nursing practice shall include both the conduct and utilization of clinical research.

XI.a. *Supporting Standard*: The critical care nurse shall conduct and utilize research independently and/or in collaboration with others. Such activities should reflect:

- current knowledge of clinical research in one's field of practice

- an awareness of one's strengths and limitations in various aspects of the research process

- support and encouragement of nursing colleagues who are engaged in clinical research

- respect for a variety of types of research efforts, each of which can further the development of nursing knowledge

XI.b. *Supporting Standard*: The critical care nurse shall facilitate current and future clinical research through the consistent and accurate recording of data related to the patient's condition and nursing care provided.

XI.c. *Supporting Standard*: The critical care nurse shall implement changes in clinical practice only when the safety and efficacy of the new practice have been established through an adequate research base and systematic investigation. Such changes must be accompanied by a written policy change and incorporation into an ongoing evaluation process.

XI.d. *Supporting Standard*: The critical care nurse shall disseminate the findings of research to colleagues from nursing and other disciplines.

XI.e. *Supporting Standard*: The critical care nurse shall determine the potential hazards and benefits related to research involving subjects for whom she/he is responsible, including patients, family or significant others, and personnel.

XI.f. *Supporting Standard*: The critical care nurse shall act to protect the rights of human subjects, including:

- the right to privacy and confidentiality

- the right to voluntary and informed consent without coercion

- the right to freedom from mental and emotional harm

- the right to know any potential harm or benefits related to participation in the research

- the right to refuse to participate in or to withdraw from a study without fearing reprisal or jeopardizing care

XI.g. *Supporting Standard*: The critical care nurse shall be cognizant of and utilize when necessary the mechanisms available to address violation of the rights of human subjects.

XII. Comprehensive Standard: The critical care nurse shall ensure the delivery of safe nursing care to patients, being cognizant of the various "causes of action" for which the nurse may be liable.

XII.a. *Supporting Standard*: Patients shall be fully advised in advance of all nursing and/or medical procedures to which they are subjected, signing a written informed consent when required.

- Related causes of action:

  Assault: An intentional act which places the victim in apprehension of injury.

  Battery: Intentional harmful or offensive touching without consent of victim.

XII.b. *Supporting Standard*: Patients shall be allowed freedom of movement within their hospital room and are allowed to discharge themselves from the hospital.

- Related causes of action:

  False imprisonment: An intentional act which results in the victim's confinement within boundaries set by a wrongful party.

XII.c. *Supporting Standard*: Patients shall receive nursing care in accordance with good nursing practice and those policies specifically established by the hospital.

- Related causes of action:

  Negligence: A breach of duty of care which proximately causes injury to victim. Malpractice is the negligence of a professional.

  Required elements of negligence:

  1. Duty of care (e.g., to perform nursing functions according to nursing policy manual)

  2. Departure from duty (nurse fails to act in accordance with policy)

  3. Damages resulted to the patient (patient suffers from some loss)

  4. Causal connection between the departure and injury, which can be demonstrated (patient injured because nurse failed to adhere to nursing policy)

XII.d. *Supporting Standard*: Patients shall be assured that any medical information will be shared only with health professionals treating the patient and that any other communication is restricted or occurs only with the consent of the patient.

• Related causes of action:

Defamation: Invasion of the victim's interest in reputation and good name by a wrongful party intentionally communicating the matter to a third party (libel is defamation reduced to written or printed form; slander is oral defamation).

XII.e. *Supporting Standard*: The patient's family members shall not be subjected to:

• incorrect information concerning the patient

• careless treatment of the patient

• Related cause of action:

Infliction of mental distress: Intentional act results in subjecting the victim to an emotional shock which is demonstrated by specific injury.

XII.f. *Supporting Standard*: Patients shall be treated in a dignified manner; only those professionals directly involved in their care shall have access to their medical information, and this information will not be released or disclosed to others without patient's approval.

• Related cause of action:

Invasion of privacy: Using a victim's name or likeness for commercial use, intruding into the victim's private life, or disclosing private facts about the victim to the public.

XIII. Comprehensive Standard: The critical care unit shall be managed in a manner which assures the delivery of humane and ethical care.

XIII.a. *Supporting Standard*: The critical care unit shall have an identified set of patient rights and a mechanism established for disseminating them to patients and families.

XIII.b. *Supporting Standard*: Visiting policies shall be developed which are based on individualized patient/family needs with consideration of effective unit functioning.

XIII.c. *Supporting Standard*: Policies shall be established to assure that patients and families participate in the decision making related to care.

XIII.d. *Supporting Standard*: A mechanism shall be established for identification and resolution of ethical issues related to the care of the critically ill.

BIBLIOGRAPHY

Alspach, J. G. (1982). *Educational Process in Critical Care Nursing.* St. Louis: C. V. Mosby.

Alspach, J. G. (ed.) (1986). *Education Standards for Critical Care Nursing.* St. Louis: C. V. Mosby.

Alspach, J. G., & Williams, S. M. (1985). *American Association of Critical-Care Nurses Core Curriculum for Critical Care Nursing* (3rd ed.). Philadelphia: W. B. Saunders.

American Association of Critical-Care Nurses.
Collaborative Practice Model: The Organization of Human Resources in Critical Care Units. (1982). (Position Statement). Newport Beach, CA: American Association of Critical-Care Nurses.
Ethics in Critical Care Research. (1984). (Position Statement). Newport Beach, CA: American Association of Critical-Care Nurses.
Occupational Hazards in Critical Care. (1989) Newport Beach, CA: American Association of Critical-Care Nurses.
Patient Classification in Critical Care Nursing. (1986). (Position Statement). Newport Beach, CA: American Association of Critical-Care Nurses.
Required Request and Routine Inquiry: Methods to Improve the Organ and Tissue Donation Process. (1986). (Position Statement). Newport Beach, CA: American Association of Critical-Care Nurses.
Role Expectations for the Critical Care Manager. (1986). (Position Statement). Newport Beach, CA: American Association of Critical-Care Nurses.
Roles and Responsibilities of Critical Care Nurses in Organ and Tissue Transplantation. (1986). (Position Statement). Newport Beach, CA: American Association of Critical-Care Nurses.
Use of Technical Personnel in Critical Care Settings. (1983). (Position Statement). Newport Beach, CA: American Association of Critical-Care Nurses.

American Hospital Association.
Report and Recommendations of the Special Committee on AIDS/HIV Infection Policy. (1987). Chicago: American Hospital Association.

Safety Guide for Health Care Institutions. (1983). Chicago: American Hospital Association.

Values in Conflict: Resolving Ethical Issues in Hospital Care. (1985). Chicago: American Hospital Association.

American Nurses' Association.

Code for Nurses with Interpretative Statements. (1976). Kansas City, MO: American Nurses' Association.

Code of Ethics. (1985). Kansas City, MO: American Nurses' Association.

Human Rights Guidelines for Nurses in Clinical and Other Research. (1975). Kansas City, MO: American Nurses' Association.

Peer Review in Nursing Practice. (1983). Kansas City, MO: American Nurses' Association.

A Plan for the Implementation of the Standards for Nursing Practice. (1975). Kansas City, MO: American Nurses' Association.

The Scope of Nursing Practice. (1987). Kansas City, MO: American Nurses' Association.

Social Policy Statement. (1980). Kansas City, MO: American Nurses' Association.

Benesch, K., Abramson, N. S., Grenvik, A., & Meisel, A. (1986). *Medicolegal Aspects of Critical Care.* Rockville, MD: Aspen Publishers.

Berenson, A. S. (ed.). (1985). *Control of Communicable Diseases in Men* (14th ed.). Washington, DC: American Public Health Association.

Carpman, J. R., Grant, M. A., & Simmons, D. A. (1986). *Design That Cares: Planning Health Facilities for Patients and Visitors.* Chicago: American Hospital Association.

Chinn, P. L. (1986). *Ethical Issues in Nursing.* Rockville, MD: Aspen Publishers.

Compendium of Materials for Noise Control. (1980). Washington, DC: U.S. Department of Health, Education, and Welfare (Publication # 80-116).

Countrymen, K. M., & Gekas, A. B. (1980). *Development and Implementation of a Patient's Bill of Rights in Hospitals.* Chicago: American Hospital Association.

Creighton, H. (1986). *Law Every Nurse Should Know* (5th ed.). Philadelphia: W. B. Saunders.

Degner, L. F., & Beaton, J. I. (1987). *Life-Death Decisions in Health Care.* Washington, DC: Hemisphere.

Donabedian, A. (1982). *The Criteria on Standards on Quality.* Ann Arbor, MI: Health Administration Press.

Fowler, M. D., & Levine-Ariff, J. (1987). *Ethics at the Bedside: A Source Book for the Critical Care Nurse.* Philadelphia: J. B. Lippincott.

Guidelines on the Termination of Life-Sustaining Treatment and Care of the Dying. (1987). Briarcliff Manor, NY: The Hastings Center.

Hein, E. C., & Nicholson, M. J. (ed.). (1986). *Contemporary Leadership Behavior: Selected Readings* (2nd ed.). Boston: Little, Brown.

Huckaby, L. M. D. (1981). *Patient Classification: A Basis for Staffing.* New York: National League of Nursing (NLN Publication No. 20-1864).

Isolation Techniques for Use in Hospitals. (1987). Atlanta: U.S. Department of Health and Human Services, Centers for Disease Control.

Joint Commission on Accreditation of Hospitals. (1987). *Accreditation Manual for Hospitals.* Chicago: Joint Commission on Accreditation of Hospitals.

Lighting for Health Care Facilities. (1978). New York: Illuminating Engineering Society.

Meisenheimer, C. G. (1985). *Quality Assurance: A Complete Guide to Effective Programs.* Rockville, MD: Aspen Publishers.

Millar, S., Sampson, L. K., & Soukup, M., Sr. (1985). *AACN Procedure Manual for Critical Care.* Philadelphia: W. B. Saunders.

Minimum Requirements of Construction and Equipment for Hospitals and Medical Facilities. (1978). Washington, DC: U.S. Department of Health, Education, and Welfare (Publication #79-14500).

National Fire Protection Association Standards. (1981). Boston: National Fire Protection Association.

Northouse, P. G., & Northouse, L. L. (1985). *Health Communication: A Handbook for Health Professionals.* Englewood Cliffs, NJ: Prentice-Hall.

Northrop, C., & Kelley, M. E. (1987). *Legal Issues in Nursing.* St. Louis: C. V. Mosby.

Polit, D., & Hungler, B. (1983). *Nursing Research: Principles and Methods* (2nd ed.). Philadelphia: J. B. Lippincott.

President's Commission for the Study of Ethical Problems in Medicine and Biomedical and Behavioral Research: A Report on the Ethical, Medical, and Legal Issues in Treatment Decisions. (1983). Washington, DC: U.S. Government Printing Office.

Scherubel, J. C., & Shaffer, F. A. (ed.). (1988). *Patients and Purse Strings II.* New York: National League of Nursing (NLN Publication No. 20-2191).

Schroeder, P. S., & Maibush, R. M. (ed.). (1984). *Nursing Quality Assurance: A Unit Based Approach.* Rockville, MD: Aspen Publishers.

Stetler, C. B., et al. (1987). "Standards for Clinically Based Nursing Research," *Journal of Nursing Administration* 17, 4, 18.

Thompson J. E., & Thompson, H. O. (1985). *Bioethical Decision Making for Nurses.* Norwalk, CT: Appleton-Century Crofts.

Underwriters Laboratories. (1977). *Standard for Safety, UL 544.* Northbrook, IL: Underwriters Laboratories.

United States Regulatory Commission. (1984). *Standards for Protection against Radiation: Code of Federal Regulations.* Washington, DC: U.S. Government Printing Office.

Williams, W. W. (1983). *Guidelines for Infection Control in Hospital Personnel.* Atlanta: U.S. Department of Health and Human Services, Centers for Disease Control.

Wilson, H. S. (1987). *Introducing Research in Nursing.* Menlo Park, CA: Addison-Wesley.

P·A·R·T IV

Implementation

AACN defines standards as statements of quality which serve as a model to facilitate and evaluate the delivery of optimal care (AACN, 1981). The standards statements provided in AACN's *Standards of Nursing Care for the Critically Ill* do not attempt, and should not be viewed, as the end point in the process of defining and assuring delivery of quality care to critically ill patients. Rather, they are presented as fundamental and prerequisite tools, a foundation with which the (desired) end of assuring that critically ill patients receive optimal care can be achieved. It is in this spirit that AACN's standards are presented as the framework needed for assuring quality in critical care nursing practice.

Implementation of standards refers to the process of integrating the concepts defined in standards statements into the daily bedside practice environment. While precise implementation mechanisms and strategies utilized will necessarily vary with differences in practice settings, the net result of implementation activities must remain centrally focused. If delivery of quality nursing care is to be assured, standards must be utilized as the basis for definition, organization, delivery, and evaluation of nursing practice. The discussion that follows addresses utilization of AACN's process standards to accomplish each of these activities.

DEFINITION OF STANDARDS-BASED CLINICAL PRACTICE

Consistent with the core value statement "The critical care nurse shall utilize the nursing process in the delivery of patient care" (page 6), AACN's process standards are organized around the five steps of the nursing process. For each step of the nursing process, a Comprehensive Standard has been defined:

I. **Data shall be collected continuously on all critically ill patients wherever they may be located.*** (Assessment)

II. **The identification of patient problems/needs and their priority shall be based upon collected data.** (Problem Identification)

III. **An appropriate plan of nursing care shall be formulated.** (Planning Care)

IV. **The plan of nursing care shall be implemented according to the priority of identified problems/needs.** (Implementing Care)

V. **The results of nursing care shall be continuously evaluated.** (Evaluating Care)

---

*Throughout the section on implementation, AACN's original standards are highlighted in boldface type.

As can clearly be seen, the comprehensive standards statements are written in broad, general terms. Therefore, for each comprehensive process standard, seven to twelve supporting standards have also been defined. Each supporting statement describes a specific component of the more general comprehensive statement. In total, the supporting standards more completely delineate the range and scope of cognitive activities referred to by the more general comprehensive standard statements. For example, there are seven supporting standards (II.a–II.g) defined for Comprehensive Standard II: **The identification of patient problems/needs and their priority shall be based upon collected data.** These seven supporting standards stipulate that **a list of actual and potential patient problems/needs will be established (II.a.), collaboration with the patient, significant others, and other health team members will occur to identify problems/needs (II.b.), collected data will be utilized to formulate hypotheses as to the etiologic bases for each identified actual or potential problem/need (II.c.),** and so on. (See Process Standards, p. 7).

By virtue of the fact that the nursing process, the universal problem-solving process in patient care, is at the core of AACN's comprehensive process standards, their relevance and applicability to virtually every practice setting is unquestionable. With the delineation of supportive standards for each comprehensive standard, the critical care practitioner has been provided the means to comprehensively and completely define the full scope of practice and responsibility in critical care nursing practice, regardless of specific practice setting.

To implement standards effectively in any clinical practice setting, however, central concepts must be fully incorporated in daily bedside interventions. Thus, the challenge of standards implementation requires that central standards concepts are translated to allow effective integration into specific patient care environments.

An example describing how the staff of one critical care unit utilized AACN's standards to functionally define quality nursing practice in their setting is provided.

Case Example: Translating Standards in a Specific Setting

Although committed to consistent delivery of quality care, the nursing staff of a busy mixed medical surgical intensive care unit were frustrated and overwhelmed by the thought of trying to define and delineate not only everything they knew and did, but also everything they thought they should know and do in providing quality bedside care to their varied patient population. Their frustration was heightened by the knowledge that increasing consumer and regulatory emphasis on quality assurance had resulted in JCAHO mandates that nursing service standards focus on and describe a predetermined level of care that staff are expected to provide (Joint Commission on Accreditation of Healthcare Organizations, 1987).

In recognition of the fact that unit standards would necessarily and fundamentally address daily clinical practice, the unit manager utilized staff meetings to solicit volunteers for a unit standards committee. Unit clinical leaders were encouraged to participate, as were several less experienced, newer staff members. In that way, the committee had the benefit of perspectives reflective of the unit staff as a whole. The unit manager and clinical nurse specialist also became committee members; the latter assumed the responsibility for arranging meeting times and locations, and assuring that the committee had access to relevant materials from the literature, while the manager assumed responsibility for obtaining needed clerical support and assuring that the committee's work was synchronized with the institution's and Department of Nursing's philosophy. The chair of the committee, an experienced staff member who had served as a preceptor for many of the unit staff members, was elected by the group.

The committee began by discussing their beliefs and philosophy regarding nursing care of critically ill patients. They quickly came to consensus around the belief that every patient is entitled to care that recognizes, to the best of the unit's ability, patient strengths, vulnerabilities, and needs, as well as beliefs and value systems. From that consensus, the group moved quickly to adoption and reconfirmation of the idea that the nursing process needed to clearly serve as the central focus of practice in their setting. With such a focus, they felt, the problem-solving process utilized for each patient would be consistent, thus minimizing the risk of omission of individual problems or needs. Before proceeding, however, the chairperson presented a summary of the committee's deliberations at unit staff meetings. All staff members were asked to either endorse the nursing process as the problem-solving methodology to be utilized in patient care or suggest an alternative framework. In a structured voting process, the staff overwhelmingly supported the direction of the committee.

With the staff's endorsement, the clinical nurse specialist obtained samples of existing patient care standards that utilized the nursing process as a framework. In addition to AACN's *Standards for Nursing Care of the Critically Ill*, both medical and nursing diagnosis-based standardized care plans were reviewed. Even though each of the latter two formats specified activities and outcomes for the five steps of the nursing process, neither seemed to fit the unit's needs. Whether organized around medical or nursing diagnosis, the committee was concerned that utilization of the standardized care plan and outcome approach intrinsic to both these formats could place patients at risk for receiving care that lacked optimal individualization. In addition, the group was uncomfortable with any framework which defined physiologic outcomes over which nursing may have limited influence. Nonetheless, it was recognized that delineation of some of the commonly needed activities intrinsic to application of a given step of the nursing process could enhance the likelihood of consistency in care, and in addition, that outcomes would at some point need to be defined.

AACN's *Standards for Nursing Care of the Critically Ill* were thus selected to provide the framework for the committee's activities. The plan was to develop specific unit standards by reviewing each of the comprehensive and supporting process standards and delineating specific applications for their practice setting. To reinforce the link between the standards statements and specific clinical applications and interventions, a three-column format was developed. Across the top, the comprehensive standard statement was written. Vertically, down the left-hand column were listed the supporting standards. The middle column was titled "Skills/Activities." It was decided that the middle column would be utilized to delineate the specific actions needed in the practice setting to fulfill each supporting standard listed in the left column. Finally, it was decided that the right-hand column, titled "References," would list resources where explanations, reviews of physiology, or policies could be found (see Table 1).

TABLE 1

Format: Unit-Specific Standards

Comprehensive Standard:

Supporting Standards	*Skills/Activities*	*References*

The committee members began the adaptation process by reviewing all of the comprehensive and supporting process standards included in AACN's *Standards for Nursing Care of the Critically Ill.* They found that some supporting standards easily could be combined and in effect streamlined, as the concepts functionally overlapped in bedside practice in their unit. Throughout their discussions, however, the committee members were diligent to assure that each of the concepts delineated in AACN's supporting standards statements was addressed at some point in their unit-specific adaptations. An example listing of supporting standards from AACN's Comprehensive Standard I, with the adapted committee-defined unit-specific supporting standards, is provided in Table 2. As can be seen, the unit-specific adaptations for standards I.a and I.b, although worded differently, are conceptually equivalent to the similarly numbered AACN statements.

TABLE 2

Adapting Supporting Standards

AACN's Statements	Unit-Specific Statements
I.a. The critical care nurse shall collect subjective and objective data to determine the gravity of the patient's problems/needs.	I.a. The critical care nurse shall collect subjective data regarding present and past illness upon admission.
I.b. The critical care nurse shall collect subjective and objective data within a time period which reflects the gravity of the patient's problems/needs.	I.b. The critical care nurse shall collect objective data within a time frame that reflects the gravity of the patient's problems and needs.
I.c. The critical care nurse shall collect data in an organized, systematic fashion in order to assure completeness of assessment.	I.c. Same as AACN's statement.

In some cases the committee felt that the concepts delineated in AACN's supporting standards were best suited to incorporation via the "Skills/Activities" (i.e., middle) column. Among those statements were AACN's supporting standards:

I.d. **The critical care nurse shall utilize appropriate physical examination techniques.**

I.e. **The critical care nurse shall demonstrate technical competency in gathering objective data.**

I.f. **The critical care nurse shall demonstrate competency in communication skills.**

In other words, the committee decided that the three concepts of appropriate physical examination techniques, technical competence, and communication would best be addressed under the specific "Skills/Activities" heading (in the middle column) defined for another supporting standard, in this case, statement I.c. Thus, supporting standards statements addressing these three concepts were not included in the unit-specific supporting standards listing.

With completion of a working draft of comprehensive and supporting standards statements, the committee was ready to begin the project of defining specific applications for the practice setting. Each committee member was assigned the task of delineation of specific skills and activities for a single comprehensive standard and its respective supporting statements. In small groups, the committee members asked two questions: "What does (this supporting standard) statement specifically mean in our setting?" and "What "should be" with regard to skills/abilities and competencies?"

Also, as part of the development process, each subgroup asked various staff members to review and provide feedback regarding the clarity and content of the working draft. Based upon feedback received, further modifications to the wording of both the comprehensive and structure standards statements were made. For example, because the committee was addressing its specific nursing unit, Comprehensive Standard I was modified to read: "A comprehensive and dynamic data base will be maintained on all patients admitted to the Critical Care Unit," as opposed to "**Data shall be collected continuously on all critically ill patients wherever they may be located,**" as stated in AACN's process standards.

When the entire committee reconvened, a complete draft was assembled and the total document reviewed. The committee specifically considered and discussed unit-specific characteristics and variables such as patient population and mix; staff experience, expertise, and skill mix; facility characteristics; technical capabilities; staffing patterns (turnover, temporary agency personnel use); and existing physician or other protocols. As a result, some entries in the middle column were expanded, while others were streamlined.

The group also realized that for some standards there existed constraints that, if not corrected, would preclude consistent compliance. For example, Standard II.d states "**The critical care nurse shall utilize nursing diagnoses for the actual or potential problems/needs which nurses, by virtue of education and experience, are able, responsible, and accountable to treat.**" The committee members were well aware that previous attempts to incorporate the concept of nursing diagnosis into critical care nursing practice had been met by confusion and resistance and had, as a result, been by and large unsuccessful. Nonetheless, they were committed to integration of the nursing diagnostic process into their unit's practice environment. Rather than give up or lower their commitment, they decided that issues surrounding implementation of nursing diagnosis needed thorough analysis and discussion. A plan was thus devised to raise the issue in the course of discussion of the standards document, and suggest that the staff be involved in defining strategies to address the apparent confusion and reluctance.

A second constraint identified was the fact that current documentation formats were fragmented and duplicative. Thus, without modification, existing documentation forms would not enhance the ability of the staff to efficiently record the information required by the standards addressing the patient's data base. The decision was thus made to also address this constraint as part of the review of the standards document in the staff meetings to come.

As a final check, the committee reviewed the working draft one last time. The committee specifically checked to assure that all standards statements and descriptions of skills abilities and competencies met four criteria: (1) Were all statements *clear* in intent and meaning? (2) Were all expectations *relevant* to their specific setting? (3) Were all expectations *realistic* given the patient and staff mix and identified constraints? And (4) were the expectations described by the standards *measurable*?

Once satisfied that the above criteria were met, each critical care staff member was provided a copy of the entire working standards document. The draft was deliberately reviewed at subsequent staff meetings. Throughout, feedback was requested and constraints deliberately discussed. In some cases, further modifications and clarifications were incorporated into the document.

Upon completion of the reviews, the staff were asked to endorse the document, again utilizing a structured voting process. The committee was gratified by the virtually unanimous approval of its efforts. In addition, the committee was pleased that not only were suggestions for incorporating standards into practice enthusiastically offered, but several volunteers emerged to assist with various projects including those designed to address the various constraints that had been identified.

Excerpts of the clinical practice standards developed in the situation just described can be found in Table 3.

Discussion

A number of factors contributed to the successful definition of quality clinical practice described in the situational example. One of the most fundamental of those factors was that the committee did not try to "reinvent the wheel." Because the goal was to address clinical practice, the committee built directly upon the framework provided by AACN's process standards, and by so doing, its task was one of adaptation and individualization. Thus, the project not only was based upon sound principles but was reasonable in scope as well.

A second factor contributing to success was the highly participatory nature of the process utilized. From the outset, those who knew best what is and is not effective in clinical bedside practice were deliberately involved. A comprehensive breadth of perspectives was sought for the committee by soliciting both clinical leaders and relative novices. In addition, the roles of the manager and clinical nurse specialist were specifically structured to facilitate group process and function, and to support efforts being expended. Thus, both the manager and the clinical nurse specialist effectively enhanced the likelihood of success by helping to assure that commitment to the project as well as ownership of the content remained firmly grounded in committee and other unit staff members, those for whom the impact of standards implementation would likely be most marked.

Change is implicit in standards implementation. The participatory approach utilized provides a lesson in effective application of change theory. Beginning at the point of delineating the philosophy and values to be used as the basis for the unit standards, staff were substantively involved. Early on, they were provided significant control by having the choice of either endorsing the philosophical approach of their peers or proposing an alternative course.

TABLE 3

Excerpts from Unit-Specific Standards

I. Comprehensive Standard: A comprehensive and dynamic data base will be maintained on all patients admitted to the Critical Care Unit.

Supporting Standard	Skills, Abilities, Competencies	References
I.a. The critical care nurse shall collect subjective data regarding present and past illness upon admission.	I.a–1 Subjective data base will include: *• Patient description of onset of present symptoms and treatments utilized, if any. *• Patient statement of current problem, illness • Patient review of previous illnesses, surgeries, hospitalizations • Present medications and patient statement of reasons for taking • Patient description of allergies and reactions • Review of family history of illnesses I.a–2 If patient unable to provide subjective data, family or significant others will be asked.	I.a. Refer to Admission Nursing Assessment Form.
I.b. The critical care nurse shall collect initial objective data within a time frame that reflects the gravity of the patient's problems and needs.	I.b–1 The first physiologic system to be assessed will be the one in which the primary medical problem, illness, or compromise exists.	
	I.b–2 A comprehensive, systems-based assessment will be performed and documented within 4 hours of admission. I.b–3 Previous patient records will be reviewed for relevant history within 8 hours of admission.	I.b. Refer to Nursing Procedure Manual "Admission Assessment."
I.c. The critical care nurse shall collect assessment data in an organized,	I.c–1 Assessment will be systems-based including the following: Neurosensory Respiratory Cardiac and vascular Gastrointestinal	(Continued)

TABLE 3 (cont.)

Excerpts from Unit-Specific Standards

I. Comprehensive Standard: A comprehensive and dynamic data base will be maintained on all patients admitted to the Critical Care Unit.

Supporting Standard	Skills, Abilities, Competencies	References
systematic fashion to assure completeness.	Fluid and electrolytes Endocrine	

	I.c–2 Neurosensory assessment will include:
	** Level of consciousness (LOC) will be described to include:
	    stimuli to arouse (verbal, pain)
	    behavior once aroused (commands, orientation, restless, etc.) best verbal response (appropriateness, clarity) best motor response (flaccid, withdraws to pain, posturing)
	** Pupillary response will include:
	    size (mm's) and symmetry response to light (brisk, sluggish, nonreactive) eye position and movement (asymmetric gaze, nystagmus, etc.)
	** Muscle tone will be described to include:
	    spontaneous, or to command, movement of all 4 extremities (paralysis, plegia), deep tendon reflexes (symmetry, speed), presence of Babinski, clonus
	• Sensation
	    note areas of altered or absent sensation
	** Intracranial pressure
	    note precipitating events with elevations
		Refer to Critical Care Flow Sheet. Refer to "Clinical Assessment of The Neurologic System," in *Core Curriculum for Critical Care Nursing,* 3rd ed., Alspach, J., and Williams, S. (eds.), 1985. Refer to Critical Care Procedure Manual: "Neurologic Assessment."

	I.c–3 Respiratory assessment will include: ** Airway patency (note snoring, retractions, stridor, wheeze, etc.) ** Respiratory rate ** Chest excursion (depth of ventilation) • Cough (productive vs. nonproductive, including nature of secretions) ** Auscultation (note rales, wheeze, rhonchi, decreased or diminished breath sounds, friction rub) • Analysis of arterial blood gas (able to recognize hypoxemia, respiratory	Refer to "Clinical Assessment of The Pulmonary System," in *Core Curriculum for Critical Care Nursing,* 3rd ed., Alspach, J.,

TABLE 3 (cont.)

Excerpts from Unit-Specific Standards

I. Comprehensive Standard: A comprehensive and dynamic data base will be maintained on all patients admitted to the Critical Care Unit.

Supporting Standard	Skills, Abilities, Competencies	References
	acidosis and alkalosis, metabolic acidosis and alkalosis). *• Determination of need for respiratory support	and Williams, S. (eds.), 1985. Refer to Critical Care Procedure Manual: "Pulmonary Assessment."

Same Format Utilized for Remaining Systems Assessment (I.c.-4-6)

I.d. The critical care nurse shall gather pertinent psychosocial data from the patient, significant others, and other health team members.	I.d-1 Psychosocial assessment will include: • Identification of key support persons • Identification of religious preference • Description of response to illness and treatment regimes • Description of usual coping strategies I.d-2 If patient is unable to provide above data, family or significant others will be consulted.	Refer to Admission Nursing Assessment Form.
I.e. The critical care nurse shall facilitate the availability of pertinent data to all health team members.	I.e-1 Patient history will be documented in the patient record within 4 hours of admission. I.e-2 Admission assessment will be documented in the record within 4 hours of admission. I.e-3 Serial assessments will be documented at 2-hour intervals (see I.f) I.e-4 Summary notes will be documented every 8 hours.	
I.f. The critical care nurse shall revise the data base as new information is available.	I.f-1 Serial assessments will be performed as dictated by the patient's condition or at a minimum of every 2 hours. I.f-2 Serial assessments will be systems-based and include at a minimum the asterisked (*) components listed under each of the system's assessment parameters. I.f-3 Summary notes will describe pertinent changes, trends in assessment data base, as well as patient response to both the medical and nursing treatment plan.	

Furthermore, throughout the process, staff feedback was sought, encouraged, and, whenever appropriate, incorporated into the working document. During the final series of staff meetings, the highly participatory tone was as evident as it had been in the beginning. It should not be surprising that the final document not only met little resistance, but in fact served to generate enthusiasm for further related projects.

Key steps involved in utilizing AACN's process standards to functionally define quality clinical practice in the case example just cited are summarized in Table 4.

TABLE 4

Definition of Quality Clinical Practice Utilizing AACN's Process Standards

Step	Rationale/Discussion
1. Solicit a committee fully representative of staff perspectives.	1. Staff members are most directly involved in patient care on a consistent basis. A realistic, effective product requires that perspectives of staff at various levels of expertise and experience are considered in the development process.
2. Assure committee support to perform the work of unit standards development.	2. Access to relevant resources (literature, clinical specialists) and clerical support, as well as congruence with institutional and department philosophy, need to be assured.
3. Reaffirm the role of the nursing process as the central problem solving framework for addressing patient problems/needs.	3. The nursing process is the fundamental problem-solving methodology in nursing care. Development of standards that reinforce and facilitate consistent application of each step of the nursing process optimizes the likelihood that nursing care will be individualized based upon presenting problems and needs.
4. Review AACN's comprehensive and supporting standards. Adapt and modify to reflect bedside practice.	4. Precise wording and organization of supporting and comprehensive statements can be adapted to match unit-specific needs provided central concepts contained in AACN's statements remain intact and are reflected somewhere in the document.
5. Develop a format to be used consistently in the development and implementation of unit standards.	5. A three-column format (see Table 1) is recommended, as it serves to visually reinforce the link between standards concepts and related nursing activities and interventions.

TABLE 4 (cont.)

Definition of Quality Clinical Practice Utilizing AACN's Process Standards

Step	Rationale/Discussion
6. Translate unit-specific supporting standards into specific activities and competencies by asking: a. What does this supporting standard statement mean in this setting? b. What skills, activities, and competencies should occur to meet this standard?	6. Considerations in this process need to include: – patient population – staff experience, expertise, and skill mix – staffing considerations (turnover, agency personnel) – technical, equipment, and facility characteristics
7. Address both real and potential constraints to compliance. Develop strategies to address constraints.	7. Proactive identification of constraints to standards-based practice allows for analysis and development of specific strategies either to correct constraints or to lessen their impact.
8. Review unit-specific standards to assure they are: a. clear in intent and meaning b. relevant to the setting c. realistic in light of patient and staff mix and identified constraints d. measurable in some way	8. Consistent compliance requires not only that expectations are clearly understood, but in addition, that expectations are meaningful and possible in daily practice. Similarly, standards compliance can only be evaluated if defined expectation can be tangibly and objectively assessed.

ORGANIZATION AND DELIVERY OF STANDARDS-BASED CLINICAL PRACTICE

Organizing and delivering standards-based clinical practice involves the development of mechanisms to integrate standards into daily practice. The preceding section, "Definition of Standards-Based Clinical Practice," dealt extensively with the first step of this integration process, that is, individualizing standards statements and concepts for a given practice setting. In the discussion that follows, three mechanisms to integrate standards into practice (standards-based orientation, standards-based job description, and standards-based evaluation) are presented. All three discussions build upon the example and methodology discussed in the first section, "Definition of Standards-Based Clinical Practice." Throughout, the three-column format, which was developed to enhance clear visualization of the link between a given standards statement and the specific activities and interventions indicated, serves as the starting point. (Refer to Tables 1 and 3.)

Standards-Based Orientation

A tool for new personnel orientation can easily be developed by merely replacing the right-hand column (titled "References") in Table 1 with two new columns headed "Validation" and "Comments," as depicted in Table 5. By so doing, unit standards drive the content to be covered during the orientation period.

With such a tool, new personnel are aware of the content, skills, and competencies that must be reviewed and mastered during the orientation period. In addition, staff members assisting or coordinating the process are provided a consistent framework from which to work. As a result, there is less chance of duplication and fragmentation, and overall, the process is more efficient.

Completion of the right-hand columns can be handled in a variety of ways. In some settings it may be most expedient to have designated preceptors or education coordinators initial and date the validation column once new personnel have demonstrated understanding and/or competence of a given section of activities in the middle column. In other settings a clinical nurse specialist or other staff resources may be designated to validate new personnel competence in or for those specific sections of the unit standards where their expertise is recognized throughout the unit. While in still others, new personnel may be assigned the responsibility of independent review of the orientation tool and validation of their own competency. Regardless of the precise manner in which the validation process is handled, the "Comments" column is utilized to record relevant observations and to designate areas of needed follow-up, reevaluation, or strength.

Several advantages are to be gained from utilization of a standards-based orientation tool as described. First, this approach tends to acknowledge past

TABLE 5

Format: Standards-Based Orientation Tool

Comprehensive Standard:

Supporting Standards	Skills/Activities	Validation	Comments

experience and expertise of staff new to the unit but well versed in critical care nursing practice, through early identification and recognition of already present skills. These personnel are thus free to utilize the orientation period to concentrate upon specific procedures, protocols, and idiosyncrasies of new practice settings rather than be forced to repeat previously mastered knowledge and competencies. Second, for new staff, such a tool provides rapid identification of priority topics for the curriculum of any needed classroom or didactic sessions. Similarly, curricula for new graduate residency programs can be expediently and comprehensively defined, while simultaneously providing both instructors/preceptors and participants an individualized, objective tool for immediate and specific feedback.

Standards-Based Job Description

Mandates by JCAHO, as well as those in many states, stipulate the need for a link between position descriptions and job/role expectations. Too often, links are obscure, and as a result, potential staff members, even after review of position descriptions, have only a general idea of what will be expected should they accept a position in a new setting.

With development of unit-specific standards, delineation of position descriptions clearly linked to role expectations is an easy task. Where duties and responsibilities need to be recorded, the unit-specific comprehensive standards and their respective supporting standards need only be listed in outline form. In that way, position descriptions are at once relevant and comprehensive. Should potential staff members desire further clarification, the full unit-specific standards document could be supplied. Under such circumstances, there can be little confusion over unit expectations and practices. As a result, the likelihood of future, subsequent misunderstandings regarding the nature and scope of expectations is extremely small.

Besides meeting regulatory requirements, defining position descriptions in such a way may provide an additional benefit. In what has clearly become a "buyer's market" for critical care nurses, particularly those with expertise and experience, being in a position to prospectively provide evidence that dimensions of practice are clearly delineated may in fact attract prospective staff members. Clearly, potential staff members have less reason to fear future surprises related to undefined, unclear role expectations than would be the case if position descriptions cannot be definitely linked to practice requirements.

Standards-Based Evaluation

Unit-specific standards are ideally suited to serve as the basis for consistent, objective evaluation of performance. A tool to delineate evaluation criteria for each supporting standard can easily be devised by modifying the original three-column format of Table 1. For performance appraisal purposes, the right-hand column (titled "References") in Table 1, is retitled "Evaluation Criteria," as depicted in Table 6. Then, in the newly titled column, specific measures utilized to evaluate proficiency with regard to the skills/activities defined for each supporting standard are listed. In this way, performance criteria can be clearly and directly linked to the unit-specific definition of professional practice as delineated by the comprehensive and supporting standards statements.

This format is also well suited to the development of leveled evaluation criteria to reflect various degrees of proficiency for the skills/activities related to any given supporting standard or group of supporting standards. For example, Standard IV.d states: **The critical care nurse shall integrate current scientific knowledge with technical and psychomotor competency** (p. 11). Examples of performance criteria for three levels of proficiency could be defined as follows:

1. To fully meet unit standards, the criterion could state "demonstrates independent performance of technical aspects of care as described in the unit procedure manual."

2. For exceeding unit standards, the criterion could state "effectively adapts procedures in unusual or nonroutine circumstances and assures communication of adaptations through verbal and written means such as care plan or protocol."

3. To reflect an even higher level of proficiency, the criterion could state "initiates development and implementation of new procedures or protocols in response to changing treatment regimes or for the purpose of enhancing effectiveness or efficiency."

Through delineation of such standards-based evaluation criteria, several advantages can be realized. First and most directly, performance criteria are directly

TABLE 6

Format: Standards-Based Evaluation Tool

Comprehensive Standard:

Supporting Standards	Skills/Activities	Evaluation Criteria

linked to defined and objective clinical expectations. As a result, the likelihood of inconsistent or incomplete assessment of performance is minimized. Second, through delineation of clear measurement parameters for performance, staff are provided guideposts against which they can assess their individual strengths and/or areas of needed attention. Evaluation conferences are therefore less likely to be associated with completely unexpected feedback regarding performance. Furthermore, the possibility that performance evaluations will be overly subjective is minimized, and should differences of opinion occur regarding proficiency with respect to a given performance expectation, the standards statements themselves provide clear direction for gathering the type of documentation needed to substantiate differing perspectives.

A final benefit associated with defining criteria for different levels of proficiency is that it provides a mechanism to recognize and reward exemplary performance. Proficiency rewards can be monetary, for instance utilizing the clinical level described in the evaluation as the basis for compensation adjustments or merit bonuses, or nonfinancial, such as designation of various levels of clinical practitioners and notation of respective levels on staff members' name tags. Regardless of the form of reward or type of incentive involved, objective means to recognize clinical proficiency afford staff the opportunity to grow clinically and be rewarded for their efforts.

Standards-Based Clinical Ladder

Even though AACN's *Standards for Nursing Care of the Critically Ill* provide a framework for critical care nursing practice, the nursing process foundation utilized allows ready adaptation to other acute care practice settings as well. In the institution cited earlier (see "Case Example: Translating Standards in a Specific Setting," page 49), the decision was made to develop unit-based standards for all acute care units, utilizing the same approach and methodology used by the staff of the intensive care unit. Additionally, there was commitment throughout the institution to standards-based performance evaluation. Simultaneously, however, there was great interest in the development of a clinical ladder to recognize excellence in bedside practice.

In recognition of the fact that relevance to each practice setting needed to be assured if the clinical ladder was to truly recognize and reward clinical excellence, it was decided to build upon the foundation provided by each unit's specific standards. At the same time it was also recognized that the clinical ladder to be developed had to assure consistency in the degree of proficiency required to achieve a given level of recognition regardless of the practice setting.

The approach selected involved the development of a clinical ladder that described levels of proficiency based upon the degree to which unit-specific standards were utilized and applied in bedside practice. Since the staff of each unit had defined the unique skills and abilities required to meet standards for each of the steps of the nursing process, development of a clinical ladder

TABLE 7

Format: Standards-Based Clinical Ladder

I. Comprehensive Standard—A comprehensive and dynamic nursing data base (i.e., one that remains current according to patient needs) will be established and maintained for all patients admitted to the unit.

Supporting Standard	Level I Criteria (Fully Meets Standards)	Level II Criteria (Exceeds Standards)	Level III Criteria (Exemplary Performance)
I.a. The nurse will obtain a patient's history as soon as possible after admission and document within a time period which reflects the gravity of the patient's problems/needs.	Histories are complete and documented appropriately within a time-frame not to exceed the end of the shift of admission.	Guides others in collection, interpretation and documentation of data for individual patients. Expands history data base as clinically indicated.	Directs others in developing patient interviewing techniques for obtaining history and in recognizing cues indicating an expanded history is clinically indicated.
I.b. The nurse will perform a comprehensive systems-based nursing assessment.	Performs a complete, in-depth nursing assessment, recognizing abnormal/variant findings and documenting clearly, concisely and in a timely manner.	Guides others in performing timely, thorough, in-depth assessment and in determining normal vs. abnormal findings and documenting appropriately.	Reviews and analyzes unit-based assessment process and initiates appropriate changes.
I.c The nurse will perform serial assessments as dictated by the patient's condition.	Serial assessments consistently reflect asterisked material; time frame between serial evaluations is clinically appropriate.	Guides others in serial assessment, interpretation of findings, and documentation.	Reviews and analyzes unit-based assessment process and initiates appropriate changes.

TABLE 7 (cont.)

Format: Standards-Based Clinical Ladder

I. Comprehensive Standard—A comprehensive and dynamic nursing data base (i.e., one that remains current according to patient needs) will be established and maintained for all patients admitted to the unit.

Supporting Standard	Level I Criteria (Fully Meets Standards)	Level II Criteria (Exceeds Standards)	Level III Criteria (Exemplary Performance)

II. Comprehensive Standard—The nursing data base will provide the basis for the plan of nursing care.

II.a. The nurse will use the data obtained from the history and admission assessment to establish a list of nursing diagnoses/ problems for each patient.	Acurately identifies obvious and potential nursing problems for each patient. Initial problem list is present by the end of the shift of admission.	Assists others in identification of nursing problems. (Because of special knowledge and skills, can clarify nursing problems for peers and recommend approaches to care.)	Teaches nursing diagnostic problem identification skills. (Organizes and presents inservices, following through as needed to enhance learning by others.)
II.b. The nurse will use the nursing problem list to establish and maintain a nursing care plan based upon patient-centered goals.	Collaborates with patient and other health care team members to develop and maintain a comprehensive care plan. Assures problem lists are reviewed and revised as appropriate at a minimum of every 24 hours.	Guides others in developing a comprehensive care plan, (Takes the leading role in helping peers to complete relevant care plans.)	Analyzes the successful elements of individualized care plans and generalizes to other relevant patient groups. (Identifies and examines a common successful intervention and shows applicability to other patient groups.)

required only the identification of criteria describing levels of application for each supporting standard. Regardless of some differences in the specific wording of supporting standards across various units, all units addressed central concepts in some form, because all had utilized AACN's *Standards for Nursing Care of the Critically Ill* as the basis for their deliberations. Thus, all unit standards contained a supporting standard addressing the admission history; initial and serial assessments; establishment of a list of actual and potential patient problems; collaboration in problem identification with the patient, significant others, and other health team members; and so on.

A constituent committee representing all major practice settings was convened. The committee began by determining that three levels of proficiency would be developed: level 1, describing performance fully meeting unit standards; level 2, describing performance exceeding unit standards; and level 3, describing exemplary performance. The committee's task then was to define performance criteria for each supporting standard for each of the three levels. As had been the case in the development of unit-specific standards, the committee utilized a highly interactive process to accomplish its task. Throughout, the committee members reported back to their peers, requested feedback, and brought peer input back to the group.

An excerpt from the clinical ladder that the committee developed can be found in Table 7.

By utilizing unit-based standards as the foundation for the clinical ladder, the end result not only allowed relevancy and specificity across practice settings, but also simultaneously assured consistency throughout the institution. An added benefit came from the decision to utilize the clinical ladder for annual performance evaluations. By so doing, staff were not required to apply or pursue a specific proficiency designation. Rather, designations were made as part of the evaluation process. If at evaluation there existed documentation in support of a level 2 or 3 degree of proficiency, that level of proficiency was awarded. In addition, annual assessment of performance relative to unit standards was assured.

UTILIZATION OF STANDARDS TO EVALUATE NURSING CARE

Increasingly payors, clients and consumers, and regulatory agencies are addressing quality as it relates to health care service delivery. Scrutiny of all dimensions of service is intense and not likely to be temporary given the reality of limited resources, rising costs, and an aging population that is making increased demands on the health care system. More and more, these groups request, even demand, tangible objective evidence that quality services have been and will be provided. That deliverers of nursing service must be able to comprehensively and objectively assure consistent delivery of quality service is undeniable.

In the past, objective evaluative data regarding the quality of nursing care have been sparse. Often the majority of such data have been problem-oriented, reflecting not so much the maintenance of quality as the incidence of events indicating that service delivery perhaps could have been improved. In hospital nursing practice, data have typically included such things as frequency of patient falls, incidence of infections, and number of medication errors. Clearly, such data do not provide much information regarding actual bedside care delivery.

To accurately and comprehensively assess and assure quality in nursing care delivery, a multidimensional approach is needed. Not only must the process of care be evaluated, but in addition so must the structure (or environment) and the outcome of care because all three dimensions dynamically and continually interact in actual practice.

In the section that follows, standards-based evaluation of all three dimensions will be addressed.

Standards-Based Evaluation of the Process of Care

Process standards by definition delineate the "what" and "how to" in care delivery. Conceptually, evaluation of the process of care delivery is a key dimension in the quality assurance triad, because such evaluation addresses the competence or technical correctness as well as the consistency with which patient care interventions are performed.

A tool to facilitate evaluation of the process of care can be readily developed by modifying the original three-column format of Table 1. For quality assurance purposes, the right-hand column in Table 1, titled "References," is retitled "Minimum Standard," as depicted in Table 8. Then, in the

TABLE 8

Format: Standards-Based Quality Assurance Tool

Comprehensive Standard:

Supporting Standard	Skills/Activities	Minimum Standard

newly titled column, specific criteria describing acceptable levels of compliance for each supporting standard are listed.

Development of evaluative criteria involves asking, for each supporting standard, what is the minimum level of compliance needed to assure that quality care is maintained? In some cases criteria may be purely numerical, describing solely the frequency at which a given intervention or set of activities must occur. In other cases criteria may address the minimum scope or comprehensiveness of a given activity or group of interventions. For example, for the supporting standard "The nurse will collaboratively establish and maintain a comprehensive care plan utilizing patient-centered goals," evaluative criteria could easily include both numerical and qualitative components. That is, to address minimum frequency an example evaluative criterion statement could be, "A comprehensive care plan utilizing patient-centered goals will be present for 90% of the patients admitted to the unit." An evaluative criterion statement addressing the scope or comprehensiveness with which patient-centered goals are developed could state, "Goals describe what the patient will look like or be able to do as a result of therapeutic interventions, and will include a time frame within which the desired status will be achieved." Another possible evaluative criterion statement, also addressing scope or comprehensiveness, could state, "Care plans are multidisciplinary including input and role delineation for the patient, clinical pharmacists, respiratory therapy, physical and/or occupational therapy, and other health team members as appropriate."

Whether criteria are numerical or qualitative or both depends to a large extent upon priorities in and for care delivery as well as upon analysis of the risk associated with poor compliance. Referring again to the standard defining the need for a comprehensive care plan with patient-centered goals, if the care delivery priority is to assure that care plans (even those that are less than perfect) are present as much as possible, a solely numerical criterion might be utilized. If, on the other hand, the priority is to improve the quality and comprehensiveness of care plans, more qualitative criteria are more appropriate.

An excerpt from a process standard quality assurance tool can be found in Table 9.

Standards-Based Evaluation of the Care Environment

Included in AACN's *Standards for Nursing Care of the Critically Ill* are structure standards relating to the critical care environment in the broadest sense. Issues addressed include, among others, the availability of appropriate equipment and supplies, physical facility characteristics, organizational dynamics, management, credentials, staffing, protection of patients and staff from electrical or fire hazards, patient privacy, and infection control (refer to page 16).

TABLE 9

Standards-Based Quality Assurance Tool for Evaluating the Process of Care

I. Comprehensive Standard: A comprehensive and dynamic data base will be maintained on all patients admitted to the Critical Care Unit.

Supporting Standard	Skills, Abilities, Competencies	Minimum Standard
I.a. The critical care nurse shall collect subjective data regarding present and past illness upon admission.	I.a–1 Subjective data base will include: *• Patient description of onset of present symptoms and treatments utilized, if any. *• Patient statement of current problem, illness • Patient review of previous illnesses, surgeries, hospitalizations • Present medications and patient statement of reasons for taking • Patient description of allergies and reactions • Review of family history of illnesses I.a–2 If patient unable to provide subjective data, family or significant others will be asked.	I.a.1–2 Subjective data are complete and reflected in the assessment data base in no less than 80% of the records.
I.b. The critical care nurse shall collect initial objective data within a time frame that reflects the gravity of the patient's problems and needs.	I.b–1 The first physiologic system to be assessed will be the one in which the primary medical problem, illness, or compromise exists.	I.b.–1 Priority data collection is evident for the system in which the primary medical problem exists in 100% of records.
	I.b–2 A comprehensive, systems-based assessment will be performed and documented within 4 hours of admission.	I.b–2 Physical assessment data are present for all major body systems within 4 hours of admission.

(Continued)

TABLE 9 (cont.)

Standards-Based Quality Assurance Tool for Evaluating the Process of Care

I. Comprehensive Standard: A comprehensive and dynamic data base will be maintained on all patients admitted to the Critical Care Unit.

Supporting Standard	Skills, Abilities, Competencies	Minimum Standard
	I.b–3 Previous patient records will be reviewed for relevant history within 8 hours of admission.	
I.c. The critical care nurse shall collect assessment data in an organized, systematic fashion to assure completeness.	I.c–1 Assessment will be systems-based including the following: Neurosensory Respiratory Cardiac and vascular Gastrointestinal Fluid and electrolytes Endocrine	
	I.c–2 Neurosensory assessment will include: *• Level of consciousness (LOC) will be described to include: stimuli to arouse (verbal, pain) behavior once aroused (commands, orientation, restless, etc.) best verbal response (appropriateness, clarity) best motor response (flaccid, withdraws to pain, posturing) *• Pupillary response will include: size (mm's) and symmetry response to light (brisk, sluggish, nonreactive) eye position and movement (asymmetric gaze, nystagmus, etc.) *• Muscle tone will be described to include:	I.c-1–6 Systems-based assesment data are complete and present in 80% of the records.

TABLE 9 (cont.)

Standards-Based Quality Assurance Tool for Evaluating the Process of Care

I. Comprehensive Standard: A comprehensive and dynamic data base will be maintained on all patients admitted to the Critical Care Unit.

Supporting Standard	Skills, Abilities, Competencies	Minimum Standard
	spontaneous, or to command, movement of all 4 extremities (paralysis, plegia), deep tendon reflexes (symmetry, speed), presence of Babinski, clonus	
	• Sensation note areas of altered or absent sensation	
	*• Intracranial pressure note precipitating events with elevations	
	I.c–3 Respiratory assessment will include:	
	*• Airway patency (note snoring, retractions, stridor, wheeze, etc.)	
	*• Respiratory rate	
	*• Chest excursion (depth of ventilation)	
	• Cough (productive vs. nonproductive, including nature of secretions)	
	*• Auscultation (note rales, wheeze, rhonchi, decreased or diminished breath sounds, friction rub)	
	• Analysis of arterial blood gas (able to recognize hypoxemia, respiratory acidosis and alkalosis, metabolic acidosis and alkalosis).	
	*• Determination of need for respiratory support	

(Continued)

TABLE 9 (cont.)

Standards-Based Quality Assurance Tool for Evaluating the Process of Care

I. Comprehensive Standard: A comprehensive and dynamic data base will be maintained on all patients admitted to the Critical Care Unit.

Supporting Standard	Skills, Abilities, Competencies	Minimum Standard

Same Format Utilized for Remaining Systems Assessment (I.c.-4–6)

I.d. The critical care nurse shall gather pertinent psychosocial data from the patient, significant others, and other health team members.	I.d–1 Psychosocial assessment will include: • Identification of key support persons • Identification of religious preference • Description of response to illness and treatment regimes • Description of usual coping strategies I.d–2 If patient is unable to provide above data, family or significant others will be consulted.	I.d-1&2 Psychosocial data are complete and present in 80% of records.
I.e. The critical care nurse shall facilitate the availability of pertinent data to all health team members.	I.e–1 Patient history will be documented in the patient record within 4 hours of admission. I.e–2 Admission assessment will be documented in the record within 4 hours of admission. I.e–3 Serial assessments will be documented at 2-hour intervals (see I.f) I.e–4 Summary notes will be documented every 8 hours.	
I.f. The critical care nurse shall revise the data base as new information is available.	I.f–1 Serial assessments will be performed as dictated by the patient's condition or at a minimum of every 2 hours. I.f–2 Serial assessments will be systems-based and include at a minimum the asterisked (*) components listed under each of the system's assessment parameters. I.f–3 Summary notes will describe pertinent changes, trends in assessment data base, as well as patient response to both the medical and nursing treatment plan.	

To evaluate structure standards, the same approach and format (see Table 9) described in the discussion immediately preceding (addressing evaluation of the process of care) can be utilized. That is, for each supporting standard, evaluative criteria are listed in the right-hand column which define the minimum level of compliance needed to assure that the environment remains safe and supportive to therapeutic efforts. As was true in the definition of evaluative criteria for the process standards, criteria may be quantitative, qualitative, or both. An example of a quality assurance tool for structure standards is depicted in Table 10.

TABLE 10

Sample Quality Assurance Tool for Structure Standards

Comprehensive/General Standard: *The Patient Care Unit will be operated to ensure the safety of patients, families, and staff.*

Standard Statement	Skills/Activities	Minimum Standard
The nurse will recognize the potential for disease transmission and will institute appropriate measures to prevent contamination and/or transmission.	1. Hand washing between patient contacts. 2. IV solutions not to hang for more than 24 hours. 3. Inspection with documentation of status of intravenous sites every 8 hours. Site changed with evidence of inflammation. 4. Hemodynamic tubing changed every 72 hours. 5. Sterile technique for all invasive procedures. 6. Culture and sensitivity reports reviewed as processed. 7. Isolation procedures instituted in accordance with infection control policies. 8. Gloves worn during interventions likely to involve contact with body fluids. Goggles worn during procedures likely to involve splashing of body fluids.	1. Hand washing occurs after physical contact involving contaminated cases 100% of the time. 2–4. Data base reflects validation of date/time IV solutions initiated, condition of intravenous site, and validation of date/time hemodynamic tubing changed. 5. Sterile technique for indicated procedures 100% of the time. 6–7. Necessary culture isolation procedures instituted within 4 hours 100% of the time.

Standards-Based Evaluation
of the Outcome of Care

Of the three dimensions (process, structure, and outcome) of quality assessment, outcome evaluation is clearly at the center of current interest of virtually all those involved with health care delivery. It is also the area of quality assurance for which objective data are arguably least developed.

Lacking universally accepted criteria to define whether or not the result of care constitutes a quality outcome, providers of health care services have little choice but to define criteria that serve to objectively measure the impact of the care provided. It is, however, precisely because the goal of development of outcome criteria is to reflect the impact of care delivered that the task can be greatly facilitated by utilizing a standards-based framework. Since the results of care are directly related to both the structure and process elements of care delivery, the relevance and validity of any defined outcome standard is largely dependent on the degree to which the defined criteria reflect the direct impact of compliance with structure and process standards.

Development of outcome standards thus begins with a review of structure and process supporting standards statements. For each standard the goal is to define the desired end point, or impact, of care delivery as described in the (supporting standard) statement. For example, for the supporting (structure) standard "The critical care nurse will ensure that the patient's privacy is protected without compromising necessary observation or treatment," an outcome standard reflecting the desired end point could state: "There are no instances of failure to protect personal privacy reported by patients, significant others, or other health team members." Similarly, the supporting (structure) standard "The critical care nurse recognizes the potential for disease transmission and institutes appropriate preventive measures" could be reflected in an outcome standard stating: "No more than 5% of nosocomial infections could reasonably be attributed to avoidable breaks in nursing implementation of infection control techniques."

When developing outcome standards to address the effectiveness of the process of care delivery, the frame of reference must be clearly patient-centered. That is, outcome standard statements need to describe the patient status, appearance, condition, or ability that will be present if the care delivered results in the desired impact. Thus, the outcome standard "There are no adverse patient occurrences attributable to incomplete subjective data regarding present and past illness" would reflect the hoped-for impact of the supporting (process) standard "The critical care nurse shall collect subjective data regarding present and past illness upon admission." In the same way, the outcome standard "There are no adverse patient occurrences attributable to an actual or potential patient problem that was not recognized from either subjective or objective information present in the assessment data base" could be utilized to measure the impact of the supporting (process) standard "The critical care nurse shall utilize collected data to establish a list of actual or potential patient problems/needs." Finally, the evaluative statement "Patients and/or significant others accurately describe and demonstrate involvement in attainment of care plan goals" could be utilized as the outcome standard for the supporting (process) standard "The critical care nurse shall promote patient participation in implementing the plan of care."

Development of outcome standards in the manner described serves several purposes. Above all, this methodology provides for closure of the loop between the structure and process components of what has been defined as quality practice, and the end result of therapeutic intervention. Additionally, practitioners are provided the mechanisms not only to identify and respond to problem areas, but in addition to clearly set unit or service goals related to quality. Tangible data can thus be gathered proactively to demonstrate the lack of problem areas, or in other words, the maintenance of quality in service delivery. This latter aspect is becoming increasingly important as JCAHO mandates, as well as many state requirements, are increasingly looking for criterion-referenced quality assurance programs. Finally, once unit or service quality goals have been defined, they can easily be integrated into medical staff and organizational quality assurance monitors to assure truly comprehensive evaluation of care delivery at the institutional level.

CONCLUSION

Implementation of standards refers to the process of integrating central concepts defined by standards statements into the daily bedside practice environment. If delivery of quality nursing care is to be assured, standards must provide the basis for definition of practice expectations, organization and delivery of bedside care, and finally evaluation of the structure, process and outcome dimensions of nursing interventions. This chapter has described utilization of AACN's *Standards for Nursing Care of the Critically Ill* in an integrated framework that facilitates structuring and delivering quality nursing care to those experiencing critical illness.

A·P·P·E·N·D·I·X

Examples of Compliance with Individual Standards

The individual practice standards which constitute the *Standards for Nursing Care of the Critically Ill* may be attained in a variety of ways. Presented here are patient vignettes which illustrate how each standard may be achieved. The examples are independent of each other and are intended to reflect various patient situations and responses.

VALUE STATEMENT: The critical care nurse shall utilize the nursing process in the delivery of patient care.

I. **Comprehensive Standard:** Data shall be collected continuously on all critically ill patients wherever they may be located.

    I.a. Supporting Standard: The critical care nurse shall collect subjective and objective data to determine the gravity of the patient's problems/needs.

        • ECG monitoring was initiated and the rhythm strip showed sinus tachycardia with 1–2 multifocal premature ventricular beats/min. BP 150/90 mmHg left arm. Apical heart rate 130/min., irregular. Grunting respirations, 40/min, irregular and gasping, with use of accessory muscles. Breathing through pursed lips with intermittent weak nonproductive cough; oxygen per face mask at 40% FIO_2. Head of bed in full upright position. Diffuse wheezes throughout both lung fields; crackles heard bilaterally at level of scapulae and below. Patient stated in gasping breaths, "I can't catch my breath; please help me!"

        • *General Appearance:* Patient easily arousable and oriented to time, person, and place. Skin color very pale and nailbeds cyanotic. Head of bed elevated 60°.

        Cardiac Status: BP 110/70 mmHg. Heart rate 90/min. Cardiac monitoring was initiated using Modified Chest Lead 1-sinus rhythm with premature ventricular contractions occurring 10/min. Neck veins distended 8 cm above the angle of Louis. S_3 gallop at apex. Bilateral ankle edema. Dorsalis pedis and posterior tibial pulses not palpable; popliteal pulses present. Weight 197 lb on bed scale.

        Subjective Data: "I can't breathe—it must be my heart again."

    I.b. Supporting Standard: The critical care nurse shall collect subjective and objective data within a time period which reflects the gravity of the patient's problems/needs.

        • Because the patient's symptoms indicated a serious situation, the nurse gathered only the essential information within the initial 10-min period. After the patient's condition had stabilized to some degree, the nurse systematically proceeded with a thorough head-to-toe examination.

- Because the patient was so short of breath, the nurse asked the patient to alert her if his breathing became more labored, explained that he would be receiving some medications through his IV to ease his breathing, and asked briefly about allergies. Approximately 1 hour later, when the patient had considerably less dyspnea, the nurse proceeded with a complete history.

I.c. Supporting Standard: The critical care nurse shall collect data in an organized, systematic fashion to ensure completeness of assessment.

- The nurse caring for this patient found that using a head-to-toe method to gather physical findings facilitated inclusion of all parameters.

- This nurse organized the data collection by using the assessment tool provided by the hospital to ensure completeness of examination and documentation of findings.

I.d. Supporting Standard: The critical care nurse shall utilize appropriate physical examination techniques.

- The following aspects of physical examination of the respiratory system were included in examining this patient:

  Inspection: Thoracic contour; deformities; slope of ribs; use of accessory muscles; respiratory rate; respiratory rhythm; depth and ease of respiration; cyanosis (central/peripheral)—pallor

  Palpation: Tenderness/pain; fremitus

  Percussion: Diaphragmatic excursion; changes in density

  Auscultation: Quality and intensity of breath sounds; presence and location of abnormal or adventitious sounds

- Assessment of the abdomen involved the following techniques:

  Inspection: Skin—scars, dilated veins, open wounds, rashes; umbilicus—signs of inflammation, hernia; contour of abdomen; symmetry; masses; pulsations

  Auscultation: Presence or absence of bowel sounds; presence or absence of bruits

  Percussion/palpation: Liver; spleen; gastric air; pain, masses; rigidity; kidney; aorta; hernias

I.e. Supporting Standard: The critical care nurse shall demonstrate technical competency in gathering objective data.

- Before assuming direct patient care responsibility, this nurse had demonstrated competency in: applying multiple-lead cardiac monitoring; performing a 12-lead ECG; assembling the flush system for pulmonary artery and arterial lines; obtaining pulmonary artery and capillary wedge pressures; obtaining cardiac output measurements; performing physical examination techniques.

- Because of the complexity of a neurological exam, this nurse followed a hospital-developed neurological evaluation sheet. Periodic inservice sessions were scheduled to assist the nurses in maintaining these technical skills. This month's session had included: DTRs (deep tendon reflexes); pupil size and response; testing motor strength; testing cranial nerves.

I.f.   Supporting Standard: The critical care nurse shall demonstrate competency in communication skills.

- The patient's wife arrived to see her husband and was obviously upset about his hospitalization. The nurse discussed the patient's condition in terms his wife was able to understand. The nurse explained that the patient's breathing difficulties occurred because his heart was not beating as strongly as it should, and that he was receiving medication to help his heart beat more effectively. The nurse encouraged the wife to ask questions and express her concerns.

- The nurse answered family questions in a manner that reflected interest in the patient and family members as individuals. The husband was allowed the opportunity to verbalize his fears and feelings of helplessness in a nearby lounge which provided a calm, quiet environment. There, gathering data about the patient continued by using a nonthreatening approach, open-ended questions, and good listening skills.

I.g.   Supporting Standard: The critical care nurse shall gather pertinent social and psychological data from the patient, significant others, and other health team members.

- Since the nurse was unable to review the chart because the resident was writing an admission note, a summary of the patient's immediate history was obtained from the respiratory therapist who had been with the patient in the emergency room.

- Although the nurse obtained much information from the patient, the wife was interviewed to determine other information pertinent to his care. The wife described her husband as a person who "is always working" and said that he had been working long hours to get his new business going. She stated that he rarely complained of not feeling well. She expressed concern over financial problems while the patient was hospitalized.

I.h. Supporting Standard: The critical care nurse shall collect pertinent data from previous patient records.

- Unable to elicit details of the previous hospitalization, the nurse requested the patient's old chart to gain information in providing more comprehensive care and preventing complications. Specifically, the nurse looked for any information omitted on the current history and physical. Numerous remarks were found about the extreme anxiety demonstrated by patient and spouse. The nurse also learned that a niece's visits had a very calming effect for both. She jotted the phone number on the Kardex and made a note to herself to talk with the wife about calling the niece.

- The patient's wife stated that he had been very healthy all his life and had required no hospital admissions. She also stated that his annual physicals at the clinic had been normal. The nurse obtained the clinic records to collect data concerning his baseline renal function as a means of comparison during the current hospitalization.

I.i. Supporting Standard: The critical care nurse shall collaborate with other health team members to collect data.

- The nurse discussed the patient's respiratory status with the physician, respiratory therapist, and chest physical therapist, and the following decisions were made jointly: (1) arterial blood gases would be obtained 30 min after intubation, and then as needed following any major changes in vital signs and/or changes in ventilator settings; (2) the flow sheet attached to the ventilator would indicate all ventilator settings and subsequent results of arterial blood gases and vital signs; (3) tracheal aspirate would be sent for culture and sensitivity immediately and thereafter according to unit policy; and (4) a baseline 12-lead EKG was to be obtained.

- Four hours after admission to the unit, the nurse noticed that the urinary output had decreased from 60 cc/hour to 10 cc/hour. The nurse recorded this on the patient's chart and alerted the physician.

I.j. Supporting Standard: The critical care nurse shall facilitate the availability of pertinent data to all health team members.

- Flow sheets were used for continuous collection of data to record frequent vital signs, laboratory data, and treatments. The nurse not only included these routine parameters, but also revised the flow sheet to accommodate pulmonary artery, pulmonary wedge, and cardiac output studies.

- This hospital had recently installed computer terminals for clinical record keeping. The nurse entered all the observations into the computer.

I.k. Supporting Standard: The critical care nurse shall revise the data base as new information is available.

- Two hours after admission, the patient manifested increased restlessness and agitation. Changes in vital signs revealed: BP 170/100 mmHg; HR 150/min; RR 30 (ventilator rate 16/min). ECG monitor showed sinus tachycardia with 4–6 multifocal premature ventricular contractions/min. The patient was questioned to determine if he were in pain, frightened, or experiencing dyspnea. Arterial blood gases were obtained.

- Forty-eight hours after admission, the patient was oliguric and presented the following signs: BP 140/90 mmHg, up from 118/68; P 108/min, from 96; R 32/min, deep and rapid, from 21; T 99°F (rectal). He also appeared to be slightly disoriented, slow to respond to stimuli, and lethargic.

I.l. Supporting Standard: The critical care nurse shall document all pertinent data in the patient's record.

- Before shift change, the nurse reviewed the charting to ensure that all subjective and objective data had been properly recorded.

- Progress notes were written on all identified problems utilizing a summary of the flow sheet data. A complete problem list was devised so that all professionals would address problems consistently.

II. **Comprehensive Standard:** The identification of patient problems/needs and their priority shall be based upon collected data.

II.a. Supporting Standards: The critical care nurse shall utilize collected data to establish a list of actual and potential patient problems/needs.

- *Problem:* Difficulty communicating.
  Rationale: The patient was unable to talk due to the presence of the endotracheal tube. Current physical state would make written communication difficult.

- *Problem:* Increased intracranial pressure.
  Findings: Decerebrate posturing of extremities in response to painful stimuli. Pupils unequal, right 7 mm and nonreactive, left 3 mm and reactive. BP 140/80 mmHg. P 100/min. R 35/min and labored. CAT scan—skull series negative. Evidence of shifting of ventricles.
  Assessment: Increased intracranial pressure related to cerebral

contusion and edema. Possibility of intracranial hemorrhage with resulting hematoma, causing cerebral edema.

II.b. Supporting Standards: The critical care nurse shall collaborate with the patient, significant others, and other health team members in identification of problems/needs.

- The nurse asked the patient's wife if finances were a concern for them at this time. The wife indicated that they were but that the patient's brother would be of some help to them in this matter.

- The nurse asked the patient how he thought things were progressing. Frustrated with being sick, the patient angrily retorted that things were "just fine." The nurse decided that the patient perhaps had a need to ventilate his feelings, and allotted extra time to spend with him.

II.c. Supporting Standards: The critical care nurse shall utilize collected data to formulate hypotheses as to the etiologic bases for each identified actual or potential problem/need.

- *Problem:* Cardiac dysrhythmia: sinus tachycardia with premature ventricular contractions.
  Rationale: Cardiac monitor 12-lead ECG showed 4–6 multifocal premature ventricular contractions per min, possibly related to myocardial hypoxia or underlying cardiac disease.

- Troubled sleep could be occurring in relation to: noise in the ICU; anxiety about the ICU environment and his condition; a high level of anxiety and nervousness that resulted from inadequate rest; physical discomfort; and anxiety about status of girlfriend's health.

II.d. Supporting Standard: The critical care nurse shall utilize nursing diagnoses for the actual or potential problems/needs which nurses, by virtue of education and experience, are able, responsible, and accountable to treat.

- The critical care nurse selected two nursing diagnoses as being particularly relevant to the care of this patient: "alteration in nutrition" and "impaired respiratory status."

- Due to the significant chest pain experienced by the patient, the nurse identified "alteration in comfort" as a major focus for her intervention.

II.e. Supporting Standard: The critical care nurse shall establish the priority of problems/needs according to the actual/potential threat to the patient.

- The nurse immediately established that the patient's most severe problems were inadequate tissue perfusion and decreased oxygenation and their effects on various body systems.

- On the basis of the collected physical and psychosocial data, the nurse identified the following problems which were immediately life-threatening and therefore the highest priorities: hyperthermia; inadequate pulmonary ventilation; increased intracranial pressure.

II.f. Supporting Standard: The critical care nurse shall reassess the list of actual or potential problems/needs and their priority as the data base changes.

- Forty-eight hours after admission to the critical care unit, the patient's status had stabilized. Short naps and decreased work of breathing had provided some rest, and the patient was now able to communicate well using the writing pad. Although communication was not yet normal, it was satisfactory to the patient and health care team.

- It had been 6 days since the patient was admitted to the ICU. His right lung was reexpanded, and the chest tube had been discontinued. Vital signs had been stable, and he had been afebrile. The morning ECG had been normal and chest x-ray essentially unchanged. Late in the evening, the patient suddenly became dyspneic and had sharp chest pain on the left side. Chest x-ray now showed an elevated right diaphragm. The priority at this time was to evaluate the pain (i.e., rule out pulmonary embolus) and initiate appropriate treatment.

II.g. Supporting Standard: The critical care nurse shall record identified actual or potential problems/needs, indicating priority, in the patient's record.

- The initial problem list was formulated according to the priority of patient problems/needs. Subsequent problems were added to the list as they appeared and were identified.

- *Existing problems:* Poor cardiac output; lung congestion; inadequate oxygenation; poor myocardial contractility; decreased tissue perfusion; history of seizure disorder (controlled); need for education regarding disease, treatment, medication, and diet modification.
  Potential problems: Cardiac/respiratory arrest; dysrhythmias; hypoxia-induced disorientation; complications of immobility; seizures; and prolonged absence from work.

III. Comprehensive Standard: An appropriate plan of nursing care shall be formulated.

III.a. Supporting Standard: The critical care nurse shall develop the plan of care in collaboration with the patient, significant others, and health team members.

- Because of the strict fluid restriction, the nurse needed to confer daily with the dietician to make sure that the patient's preferences were included on the tray in the appropriate amounts.

- Since the physician had reported that the patient was going to surgery for stabilization of the fracture, the nurse asked one of the OR nurses to talk with the patient and family, and to help identify the patient's pre-op teaching needs.

III.b. Supporting Standard: The critical care nurse shall determine nursing interventions for each problem/need.

- To evaluate cardiac output, several assessment techniques were selected: assess P, R, BP every hour; auscultate lungs every 2 hours; record pulmonary artery reading every hour and alert physician if greater than 18 mmHg.; note color and temperature of extremities and presence/strength of peripheral pulses every hour; assess for changes in level of consciousness every hour; record accurate I & O; alert physician if urine output less than 30 cc for 2 consecutive hours; and weigh daily at 6 a.m.

- Utilizing a copy of the Standardized Care Plan for Pneumothorax as a guideline, the nurse outlined the care required specifically for this patient. The interventions regarding bronchial hygiene measures were modified so that they would apply specifically to this patient.

III.c. Supporting Standard: The critical care nurse shall incorporate interventions that communicate acceptance of the patient's beliefs, culture, religion, and socioeconomic background.

- Through consultation with the patient and her husband, it was discovered that the patient had a fear of the dark and consequently, had difficulty sleeping without a light on. Arrangements were made so that a light was kept on at night in the patient's cubicle.

- Because of the patient's reluctance to ask for pain medication as often as needed, the nurse indicated on the care plan that a pain medication, ordered on a 2–4-hour prn basis should be offered every 3 hours and before chest tube removal.

III.d. Supporting Standard: The critical care nurse shall identify areas for education of the patient and significant others.

- When talking with the patient about his medications and fluid and activity limitations prior to discharge, the nurse again discussed the relation of the fluid limit to the patient's heart failure episodes.

- The physical therapist demonstrated and explained the patient's exercises to the nursing staff and family so that the staff and brother could monitor the exercises when the physical therapist was not available. This was reflected in the care plan.

III.e. Supporting Standard: The critical care nurse shall identify appropriate goals for each problem/need in collaboration with the patient, significant others, and other health team members.

- The patient's major problem was identified as congestive heart failure (CHF) due to low cardiac output from a poorly contracting myocardium. It was decided that the major emphasis of nursing care for the first 24 hours was to minimize demands on the cardiovascular system.

- The patient-centered objective developed by the nurse was: Absence of further deterioration of level of consciousness as evidenced by: BP 100–140/50–80 mmHg; P 70–100/min, regular; T 98–100°F, rectally; R 14–22, regular; absence of seizures; and maintenance of current pupillary response.

III.f. Supporting Standard: The critical care nurse shall organize the plan to reflect the priority of identified problems/needs.

- Several problems had been identified by the nurse, who prioritized the altered pulmonary status as the primary problem since that was the most threatening to the patient's well-being at this time.

- Although the family was extremely anxious, the problem list reflected the fact that the pneumothorax was the most pressing problem. The nurse did give attention to allaying the family's anxiety while striving to stabilize the patient's respiratory status.

III.g. Supporting Standard: The critical care nurse shall revise the plan of care to reflect the patient's current status.

- After the patient's cardiac status improved sufficiently, the patient's major problem was identified as an inadequate knowledge base relative to management of CHF.

- Five days postreduction of the fractured right femur, the patient developed sinus tachycardia and a fever. A foul odor emanated from the cast. The cast was bivalved, and drainage and inflammation were observed at the operative site. The new problem and resultant nursing care implications were added to the nursing care plan and were given a high priority.

III.h. Supporting Standard: The critical care nurse shall identify activities through which care will be evaluated.

- In monitoring the nursing care, the nurse observed the outcomes of the therapies: evaluated the patient's R, P, BP, and urinary output, as well as any changes in strength of peripheral pulses; auscultated the lungs to check for rales; noted the changes in pulmonary artery pressures. Since the pulse had decreased from 120 to 108, the urine output was averaging 60 cc/hour, peripheral pulses were stronger, and the patient said he could breathe easier, the nurse assessed that improvement had occurred.

- During walking rounds at change of shift, all oncoming nurses listened to the primary nurse succinctly outline the patient's problems, the current status, and the identified interventions. Questions were asked about his progress, and one of the nurses suggested a different way to position the patient for greater comfort.

III.i. Supporting Standard: The critical care nurse shall communicate the plan to those involved in the patient's care.

- Since so many individuals were involved in this patient's care, the nurse coordinated plans for a team conference and invited the following staff: the intern, resident, pharmacist, respiratory therapist, dietician, social worker, chaplain, and the patient's evening and night nurse.

- The nurse communicated the plan of care to the other health team members via the care plan at the bedside and the progress notes in the permanent record. In addition, members of the family were kept informed since they were helping to monitor the patient's level of consciousness and were assisting in the reorientation process.

III.j. Supporting Standard: The critical care nurse shall record the plan of nursing care in the patient record.

- As new problems arose or old ones were resolved, the nurse made a SOAP note in the chart. Otherwise, at the end of each shift, a progress note on the patient's general condition was recorded.

- The nursing plan of care was initiated and kept at the bedside. At the end of the shift, the nurse charted on the progress notes and, rather than again recording all the interventions identified, wrote under the plan portion of the POMR note: "See plan of nursing care outlined on admission."

IV. Comprehensive Standard: The plan of nursing care shall be implemented according to the priority of identified problems/needs.

IV.a. Supporting Standard: The critical care nurse shall implement the plan of nursing care in collaboration with the patient, significant others, and other health team members.

• The nurse scheduled a multidisciplinary conference including the family to discuss the best approach for telling the patient about the death of his girlfriend.

• A major part of the patient's care depended on hemodialysis therapy and maintaining dietary and fluid restrictions. The nurse needed to collaborate with the hemodialysis staff in terms of scheduling treatments for the patient, as well as to plan teaching for him and his family, and to meet the psychological needs that might arise as a result of the therapy.

IV.b. Supporting Standard: The critical care nurse shall support and promote patient participation in care.

• Prior to beginning medication instruction, the nurse assessed the patient's knowledge of his drugs. He stated he was not interested in what the drug did. He would take the medication if someone could develop a schedule he could manage while at work. The nurse, the patient, and the physician worked together to develop a medication regimen.

• Although the patient was comatose and could not actively participate in her own care, her family showed considerable interest in her condition and her care. Her mother indicated she was interested in assisting with care but she was uncomfortable with bathing her daughter. The nurse suggested she comb and braid her daughter's hair daily.

IV.c. Supporting Standard: The critical care nurse shall deliver care in an organized, humanistic manner.

• The patient was to have his chest tube removed later in the morning. Since this could be a painful procedure, the nurse explained what would happen and that a small dose of analgesic would be administered. After gathering the necessary equipment, the nurse assisted in the removal of the chest tube, explaining each step of the process.

• This patient had intermittent periods of disorientation and restlessness. Since maintenance of shunt patency was imperative, the critical care nurse stabilized the cannula with a board and gauze wrap, restraining his shunt arm only after he hit the arm against the side rail and pulled on the cannula.

IV.d. Supporting Standard: The critical care nurse shall demonstrate technical and psychomotor competency in the delivery of care.

- The nurse monitored the intraventricular and arterial pressures and compared any changes in values with the overall patient status.

- The nurse carefully monitored the chest drainage, regulated the flow of the blood transfusion, and calculated the patient's blood replacement balance every hour.

IV.e. Supporting Standard: The critical care nurse shall provide care in such a way as to prevent complications and life-threatening situations.

- Since the patient was being mechanically ventilated, the nurse wanted to prevent even minimal complications associated with this intervention. Nursing care was planned to reflect: (1) prevention of airway obstruction through endotracheal suctioning and measures to reduce lung congestion; (2) maintenance of an accurate alarm system; and (3) prevention of life-threatening dysrhythmias through continuous cardiac monitoring and lidocaine bolus at bedside.

- The nurse planned the care of the patient in order of priority to deal with potentially life-threatening situations. This included: (1) prevention of cardiac arrest by decreasing the patient's acidotic and hyperkalemic states; (2) prevention of hemorrhage by stabilizing and securing the arteriovenous shunt and observation of leg dressing for bleeding; and (3) prevention of pulmonary edema by monitoring fluid balance.

IV.f. Supporting Standard: The critical care nurse shall coordinate care delivered by other health team members.

- One person must coordinate patient care to ensure that efforts are not duplicated or therapies neglected. Since nurses have the most prolonged contact with the patient, family, or significant others and other members of the health team, nurses are in a prime position to coordinate patient care activities. Coordination responsibilities include: (1) scheduling therapeutic measures to ensure optimal effectiveness and patient rest/comfort; (2) communicating all pertinent verbal and written data on an ongoing basis; (3) conducting patient conferences with appropriate health team members for communication and problem solving; and (4) continually updating the nursing care plan.

IV.g. Supporting Standard: The critical care nurse shall document interventions in the record.

- SAMPLE OF CHARTING:
  Problem: Altered pulmonary status
  Intervention: Percussion, vibration to lateral and posterior aspects right lower lobe, with patient in right side lying position with head of bed flat, followed by 20 min of postural drainage in same position. Large amount of thick rust-colored secretions suctioned via endotracheal tube. Diffuse crackles over lower lung fields bilaterally.

- TYPED INTO COMPUTER RECORDS
  8:30 a.m.—Intracranial pressure 17 torr. Decerebrate posture in response to pain. Right pupil reacts more slowly than left.
  8:45 a.m.—Intracranial pressure 19 torr. Ambued for 3 minutes. Intracranial pressure 15 torr.
  9:00 a.m.—Intracranial pressure 20 torr. Furosemide 40 mg IV given.

V.   **Comprehensive Standard:** The results of nursing care shall be continuously evaluated.

V.a.   Supporting Standard: The critical care nurse shall assure the relevance of the nursing interventions to identified patient problems/ needs.

- Since the patient's status had improved in response to the therapeutic interventions for decreased oxygenation and poor cardiac output, the nurse determined that the goals were being met. However, patient instruction regarding knowledge of his illness and medications would have to be delayed until the patient demonstrated a readiness to learn.

- With this patient's particular situation, the goal of maintaining shunt patency with inspection every 2 hours was inadequate, and another method would need to be devised.

V.b.   Supporting Standard: The critical care nurse shall collect data for evaluation within an appropriate time interval after intervention.

- Immediately after administering an IV bolus of lidocaine for 10 premature ventricular contractions/min, the nurse evaluated the patient for change in rhythm and for untoward effects of lidocaine. Although the premature ventricular contractions were abolished and the blood pressure was stable, observation continued for recurrence of dysrhythmias.

- At 2200 hours, the nurse administered morphine sulfate, 10 mg, for sharp incisional pain in lower abdomen. At 2230, the patient was observed sleeping with no restlessness. Response to pain medication was satisfactory, and this was charted.

V.c. Supporting Standard: The critical care nurse shall compare the patient's response with expected results.

- Twelve hours after beginning the bronchial hygiene regimen, the nurse examined the patient's response to the interventions. At this time, the patient's lungs remained congested, and her secretions were thick. The nurse had expected, upon auscultation, to find a decrease in secretions and crackles, but this had not occurred.

- Five days after admission to the coronary care unit, the nurse reviewed the patient's goals and nursing interventions. His weight had decreased 9 lb since admission. He felt he was able to breathe better. There was no neck vein distention. Heart rate was stable, 75–90/min, without serious dysrhythmias. Blood pressure was 120/74 mmHg. The nurse noted the patient had the expected response to therapy for congestive heart failure. Digitalization, diuretics, and fluid restriction had decreased fluid retention.

V.d. Supporting Standard: The critical care nurse shall base the evaluation on data from pertinent sources.

- The nurse reviewed the patient's progress with the physician on morning rounds. The patient had shown significant improvement, the lab results reflected normalizing values, and the lungs were clear.

- In reviewing the patient's nursing care, the head nurse consulted written records, interviewed the patient and his family, and then discussed the plan of care in a team conference. It was noted that all information obtained from these sources had been reflected in the written plan of care.

V.e. Supporting Standard: The critical care nurse shall collaborate with the patient, significant others, and health team members in the evaluation process.

- The patient indicated that she was still dyspneic after suctioning, and frequently pointed to the endotracheal tube, wanting to be suctioned. Her husband, however, felt she was a little improved because she had better skin color. In discussing this with the physician, the nurse learned that the patient's lungs were clearer on x-ray, which confirmed her assessment through examination. They speculated that the basis for continued dyspnea was the patient's extreme anxiety in spite of the fact that she had improved clinically.

- Five days after admission, the patient stated he felt much better and was breathing much more easily now. His wife reported that he was eating a little better, but that he complained of the diet being too bland.

V.f. Supporting Standard: The critical care nurse shall attempt to determine the cause of any significant differences between the patient's response and the expected response.

- In spite of indicated hydration and aggressive pulmonary care, the patient's secretions remained thick and auscultation revealed that the lungs remained congested.

- Questioning whether the patient was sufficiently hydrated to allow for easy removal of secretions, the nurse reviewed the patient's I and O status, as well as the bronchial hygiene regimen. Finding that the patient had only taken in 500 cc in the last 12 hours, the nurse hypothesized that: (1) the patient was not sufficiently hydrated to liquefy secretions; (2) the frequency of bronchial hygiene measures was inadequate; and (3) the humidification and bronchial hygiene measures were inadequately coordinated.

V.g. Supporting Standard: The critical care nurse shall review the plan of care and revise it based on the evaluation results.

- Having decided that high humidification would be helpful for mobilization of secretions, the nurse recommended the following interventions to the physician: (1) give ultrasonic nebulizer treatments for 15 min/4 hours for 2 days, then every 8 hours for 2 days; (2) administer O_2 in conjunction with high humidity; and (3) increase fluid intake to 1800 cc/24 hours—and ensure that patient achieves this intake.

- The nurse needed to observe parameters indicative of neurological deterioration: level of consciousness, pupil signs, intracranial pressure, and vital signs every 30 min until stable. Since the patient's condition had remained stable for 4 hours, the nurse changed the plan to assess the neurological signs every hour.

V.h. Supporting Standard: The critical care nurse shall document evaluation findings in the patient record.

- SAMPLE CHARTING:
  Problem: Altered pulmonary status
  Goal: Lungs clear to examination
  O: Large amount of thick rust-colored secretions suctioned per endotracheal tube. Diffuse crackles over lower posterior lung fields bilaterally.

A: Secretions remain thick and difficult to clear despite bronchial hygiene measures.

Plan: Consult with physician regarding increasing frequency of ultrasonic nebulizer; consult with physician regarding adequacy of systemic hydration; continue bronchial hygiene measures every 4 hours; reevaluate status in 12 hours.

(12 hours later)

O: Large amount of watery rust-colored secretions suctioned per endotracheal tube following bronchial hygiene measures. Right base of lungs clearer than left.

A: Secretions being mobilized; lungs clearing.

P: -Continue present bronchial hygiene regimen.
-Reassess efficacy in 12 hours.

- SAMPLE CHARTING:

Problem: Patency of arteriovenous shunt

Goal: Patient and family will be able to care for shunt.

Have the patient and his family describe how to care for the shunt; nurse observes patient and his family perform shunt care on a mannequin. Nurse observes patient and his family perform shunt care on the patient; ask the patient and his family specific questions about shunt care; and give the patient and his family a paper-and-pencil test to evaluate their knowledge of shunt care.

Assessment: The cannula was securely in position, with no sign of infection; however, the shunt was not patent. Therefore, the goal of maintaining patency was not achieved. The patient had been able to describe the routine shunt care and to perform this on a mannequin. Therefore, certain criteria of this goal have been met.